PICTURE BOOK OF HAPPY BABIES

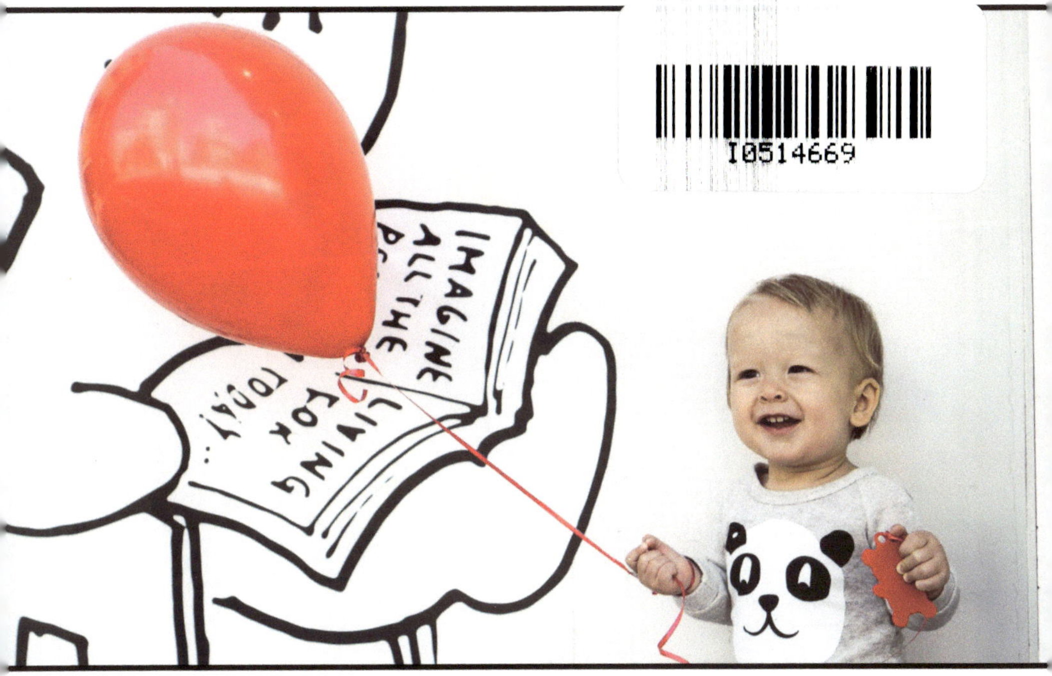

MIGHTY OAK BOOKS

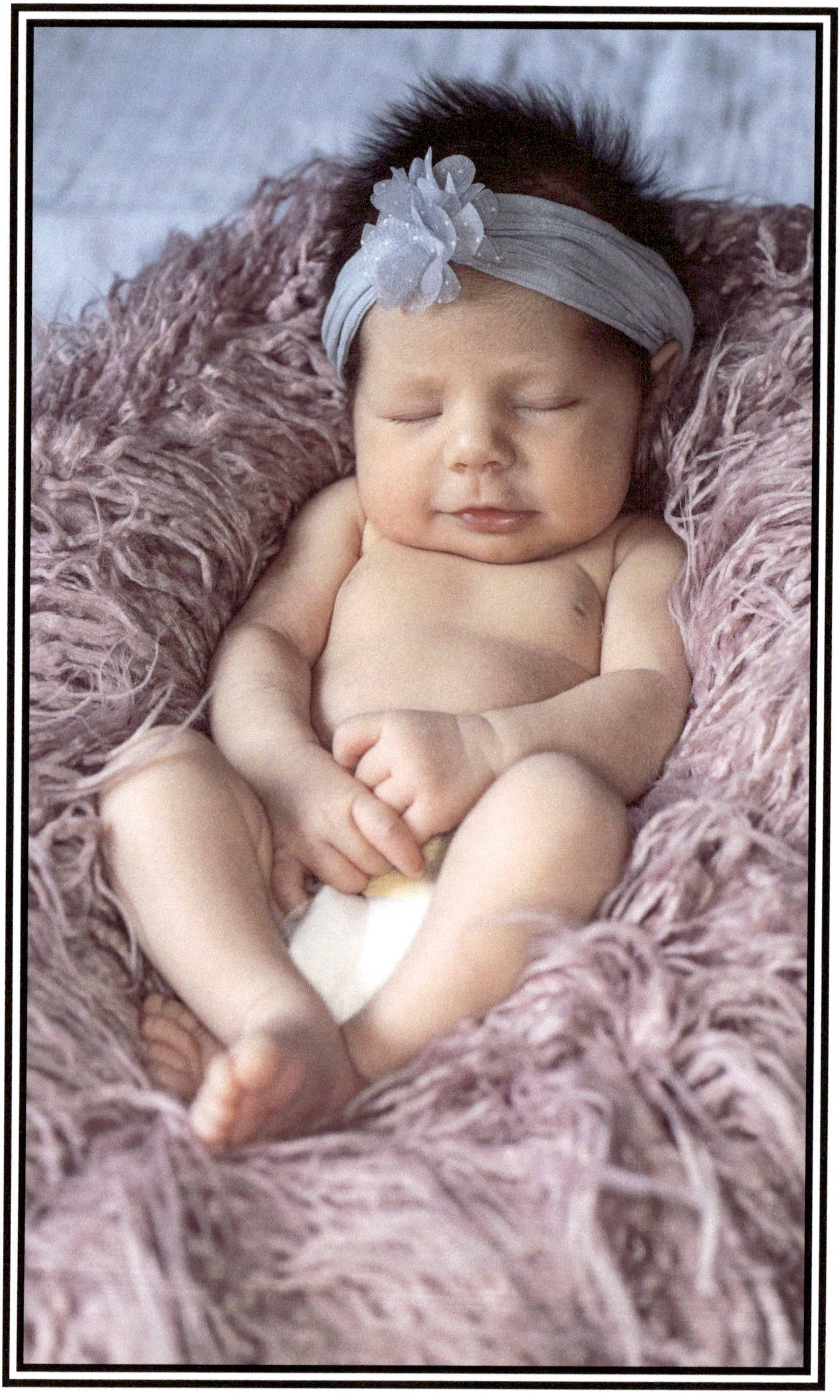

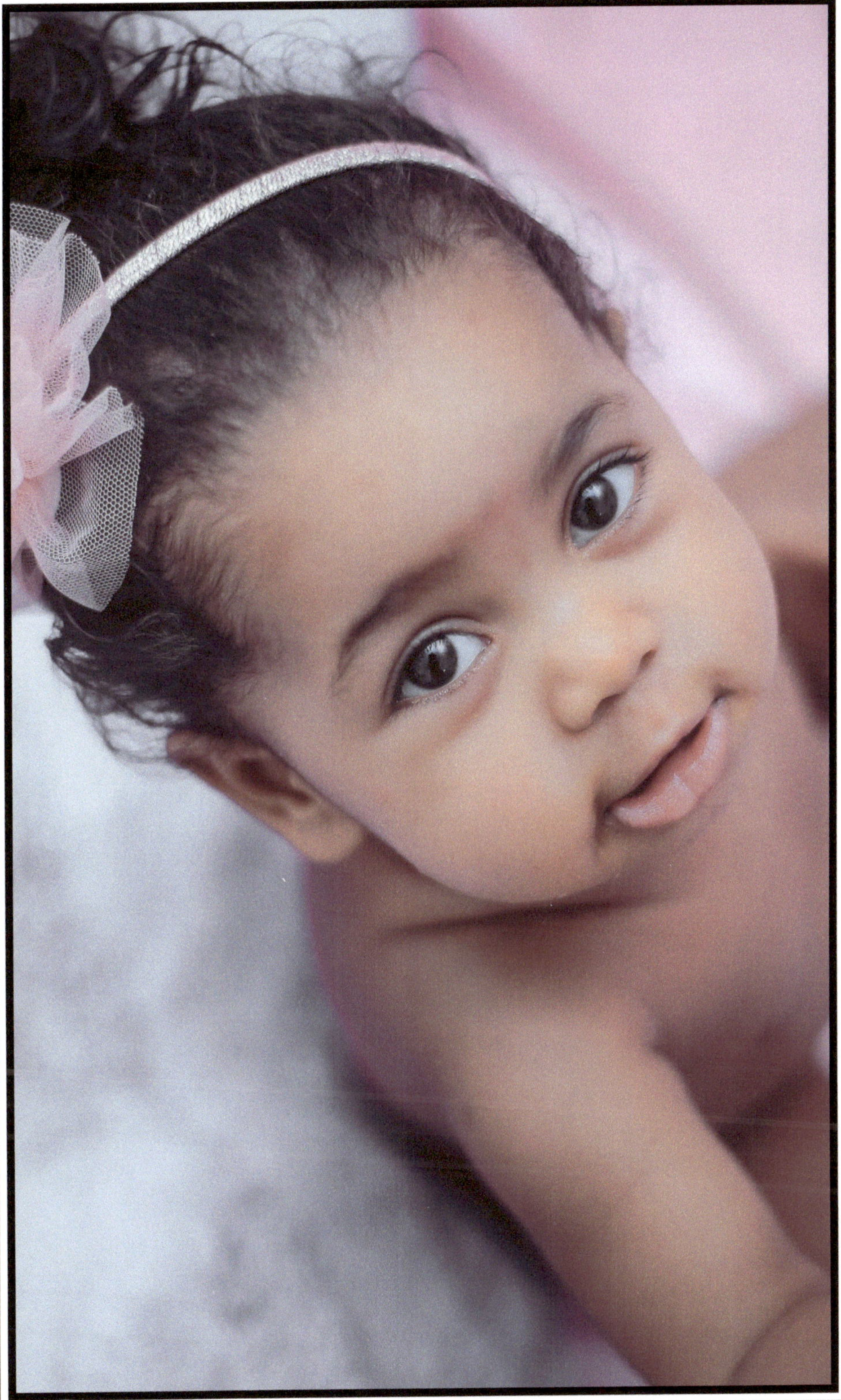

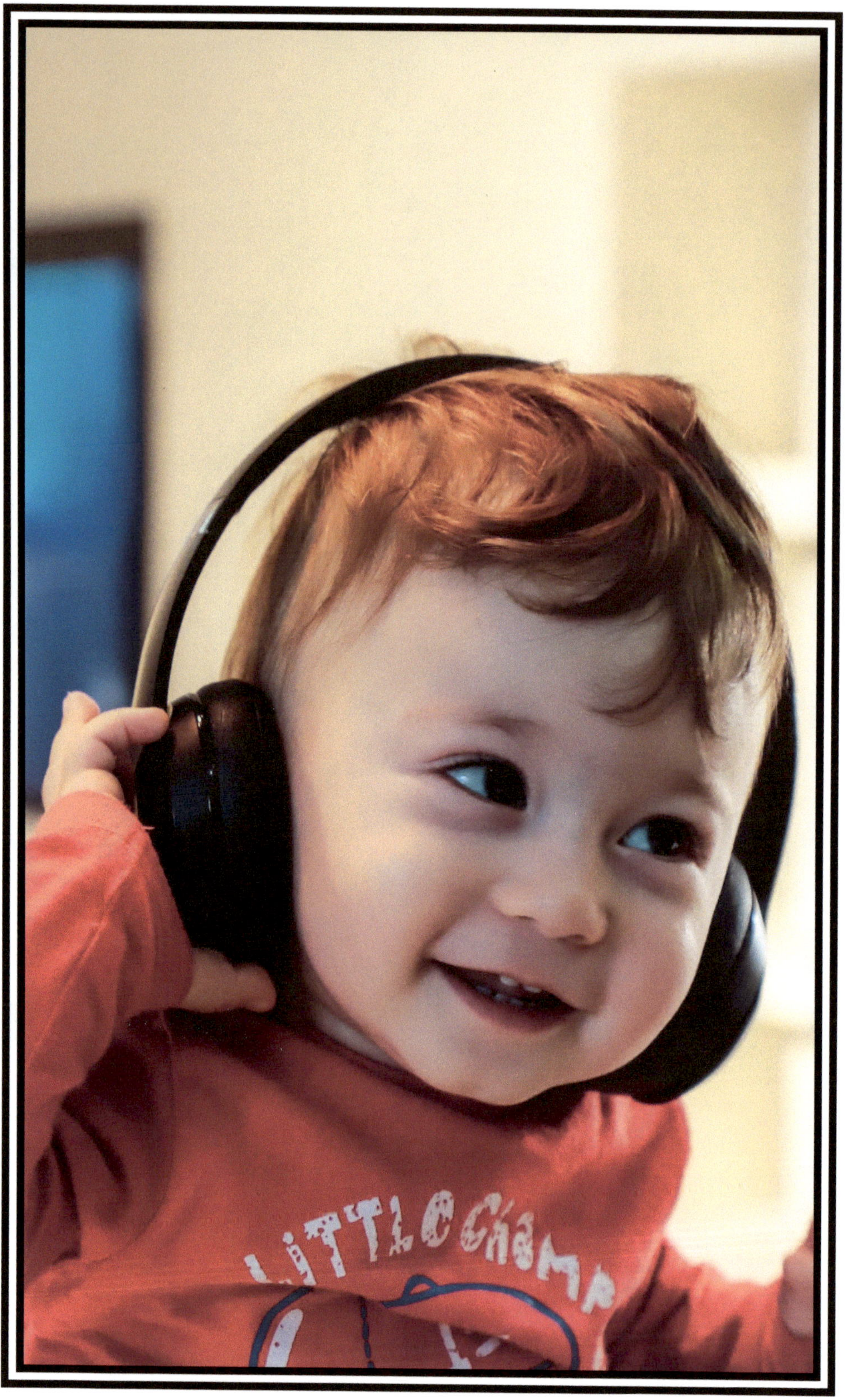
LITTLE CHAMP

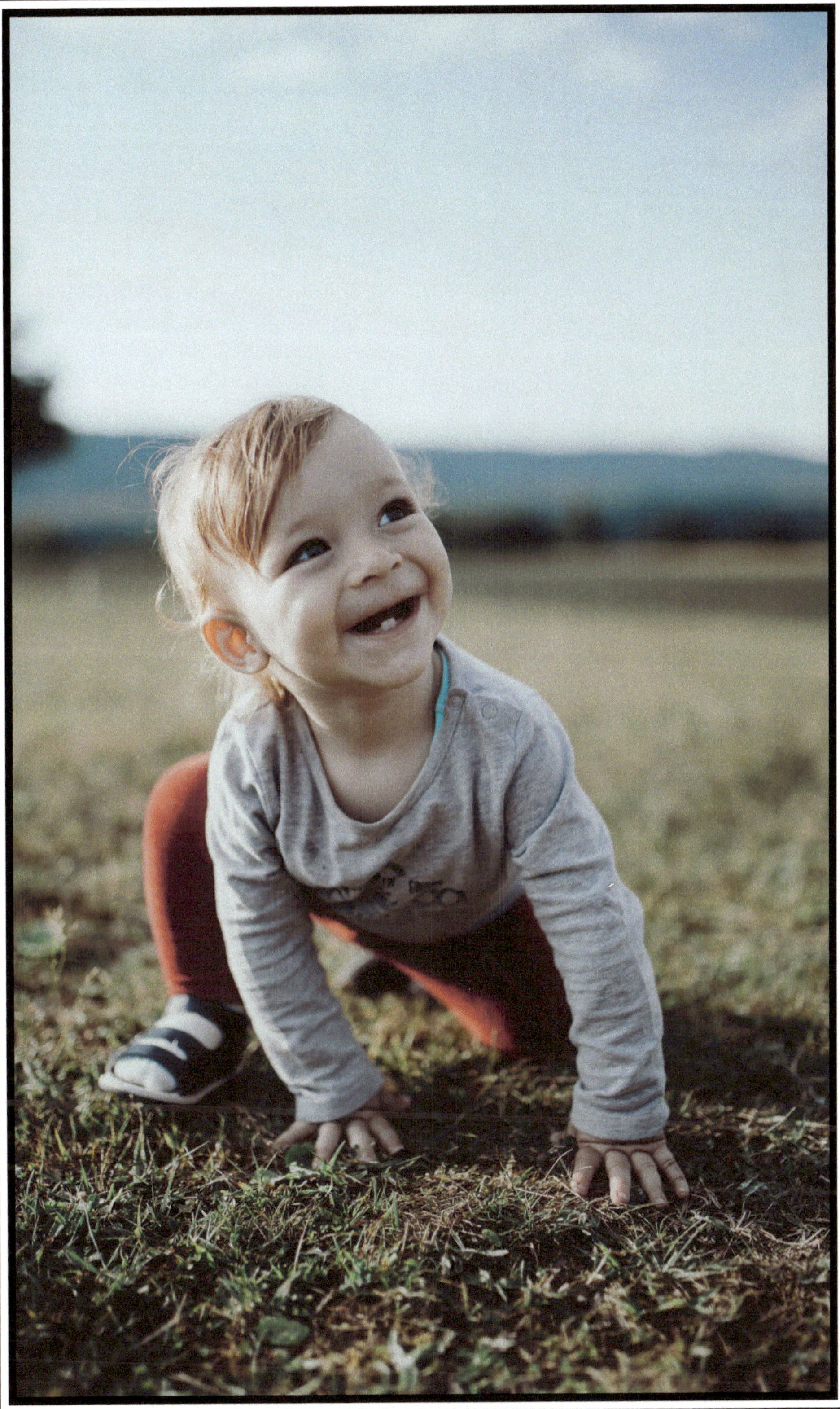

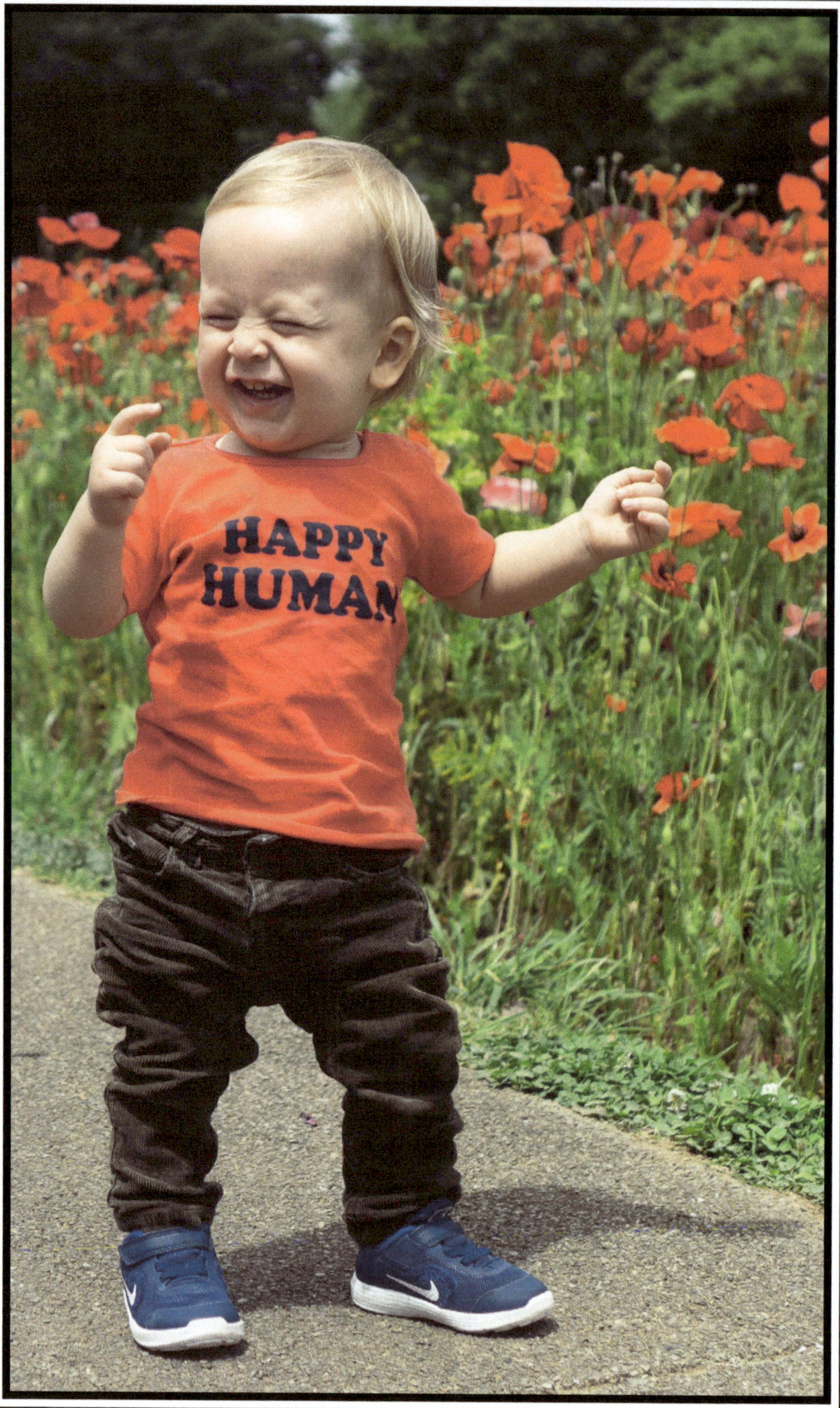
HAPPY
HUMAN

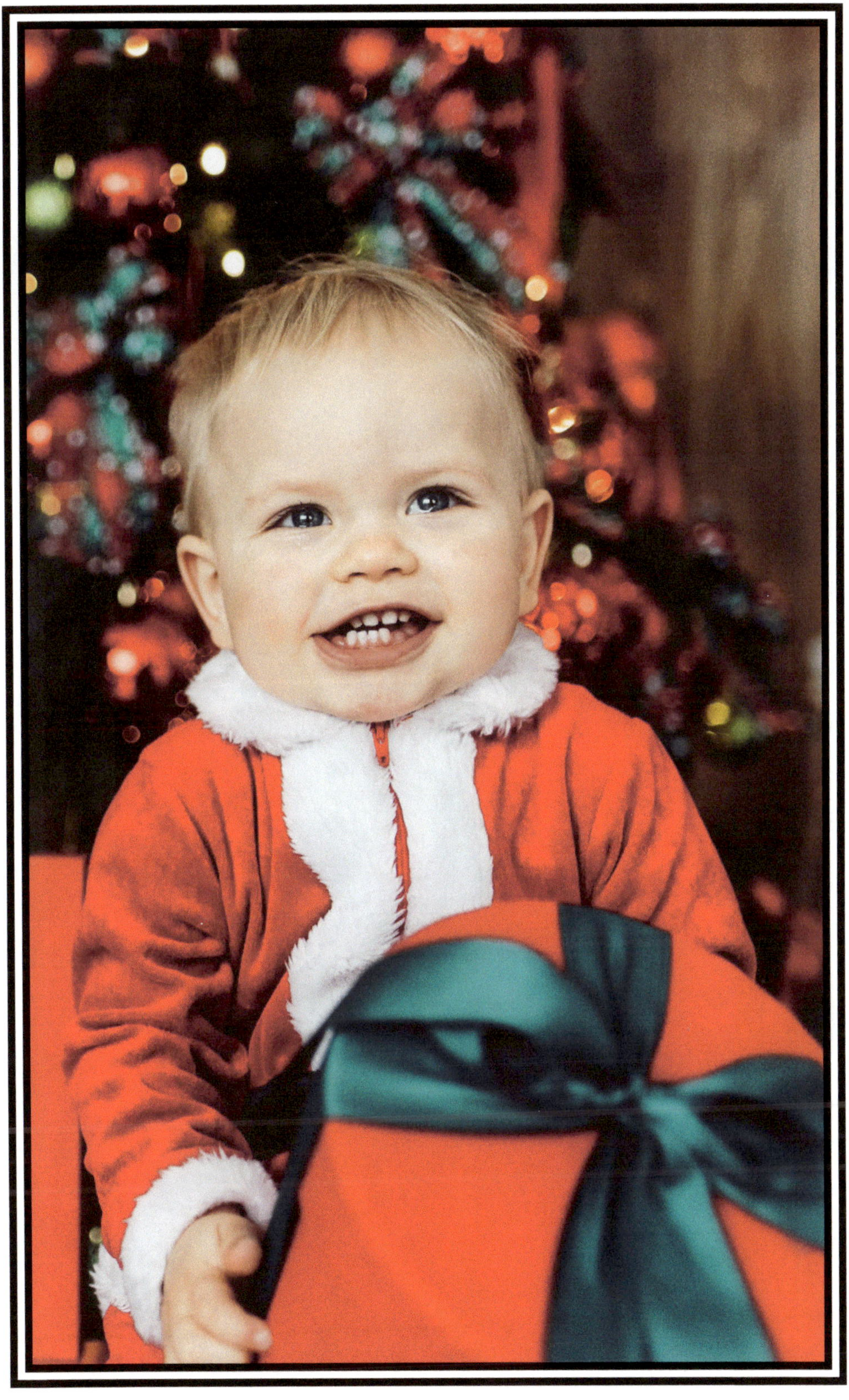

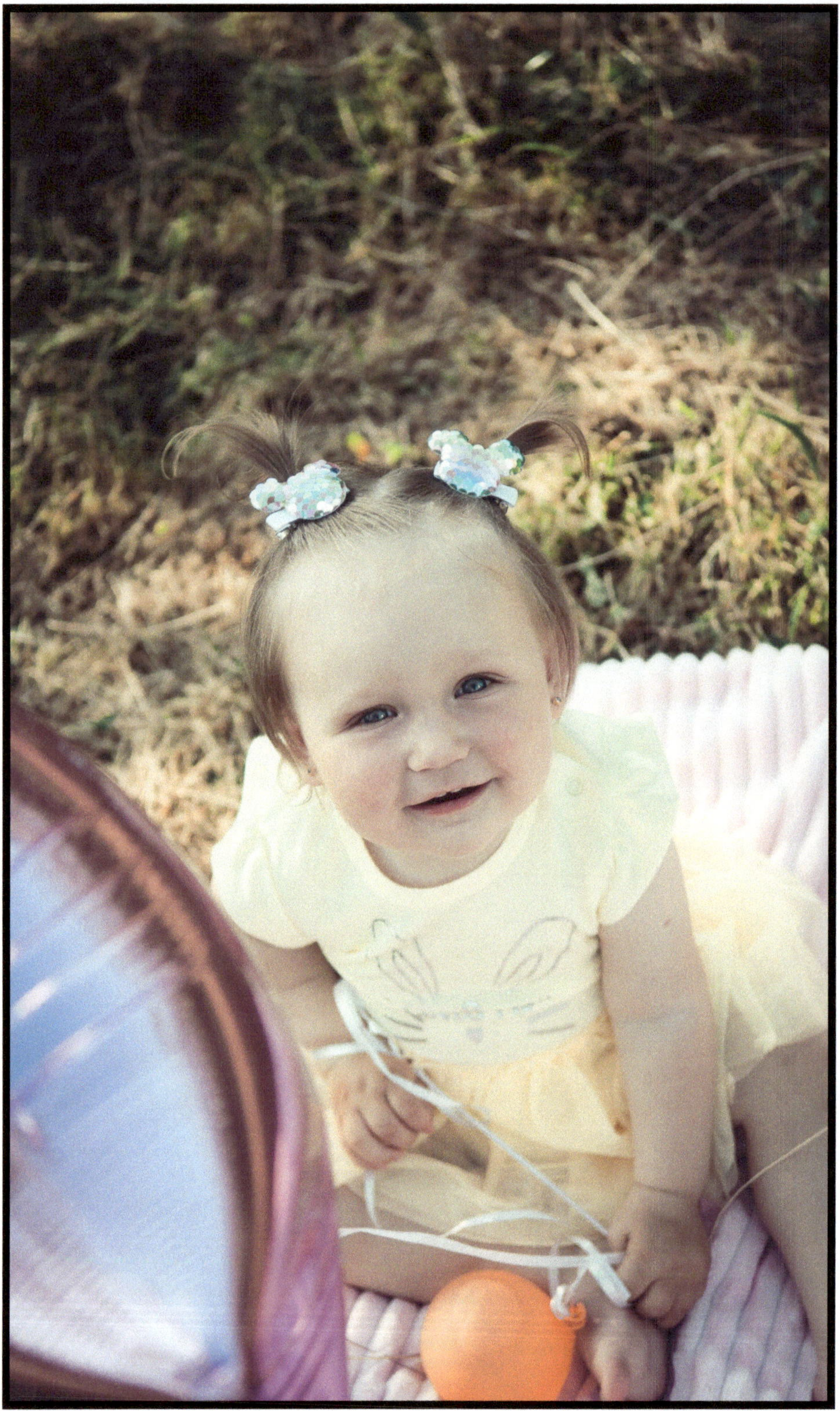

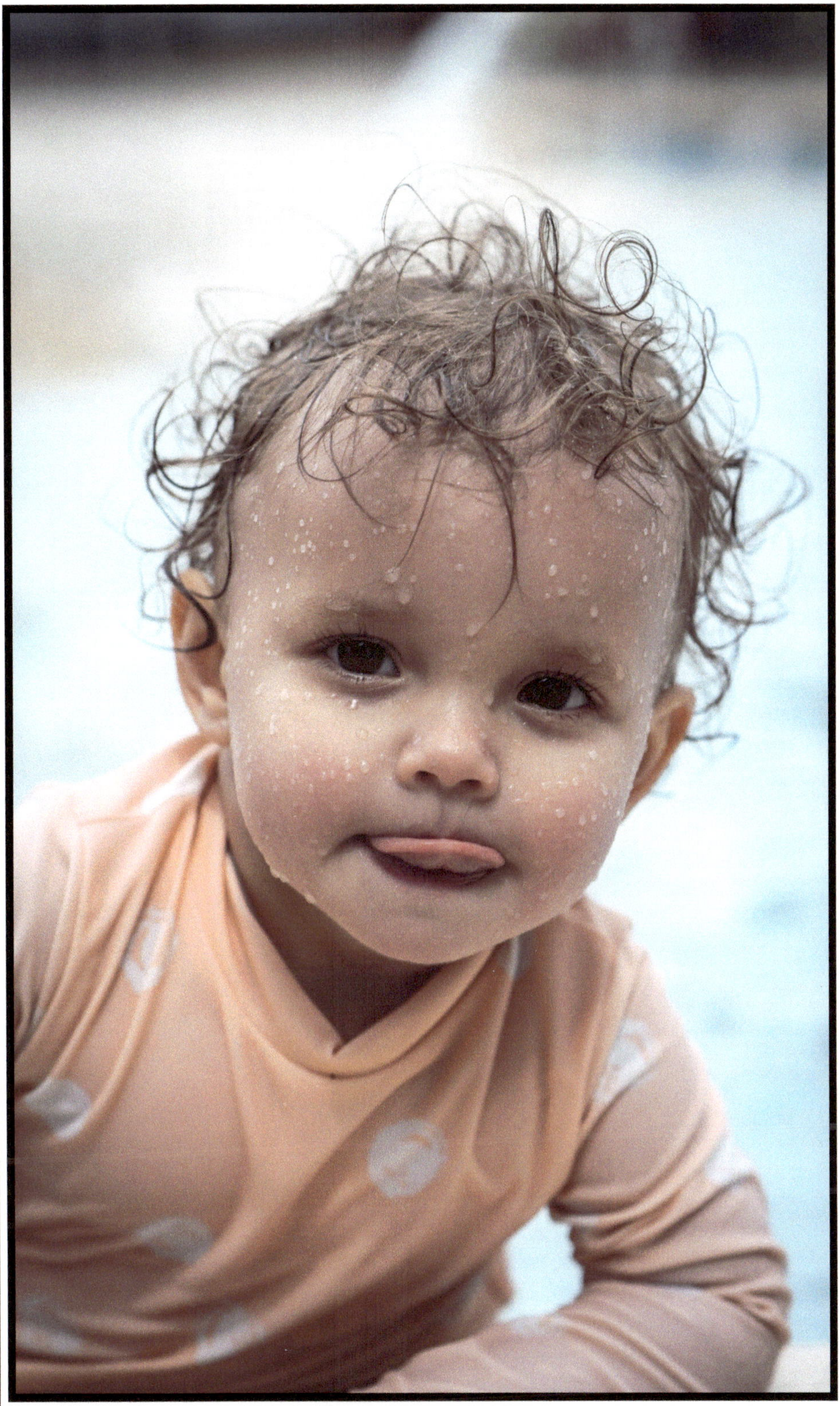

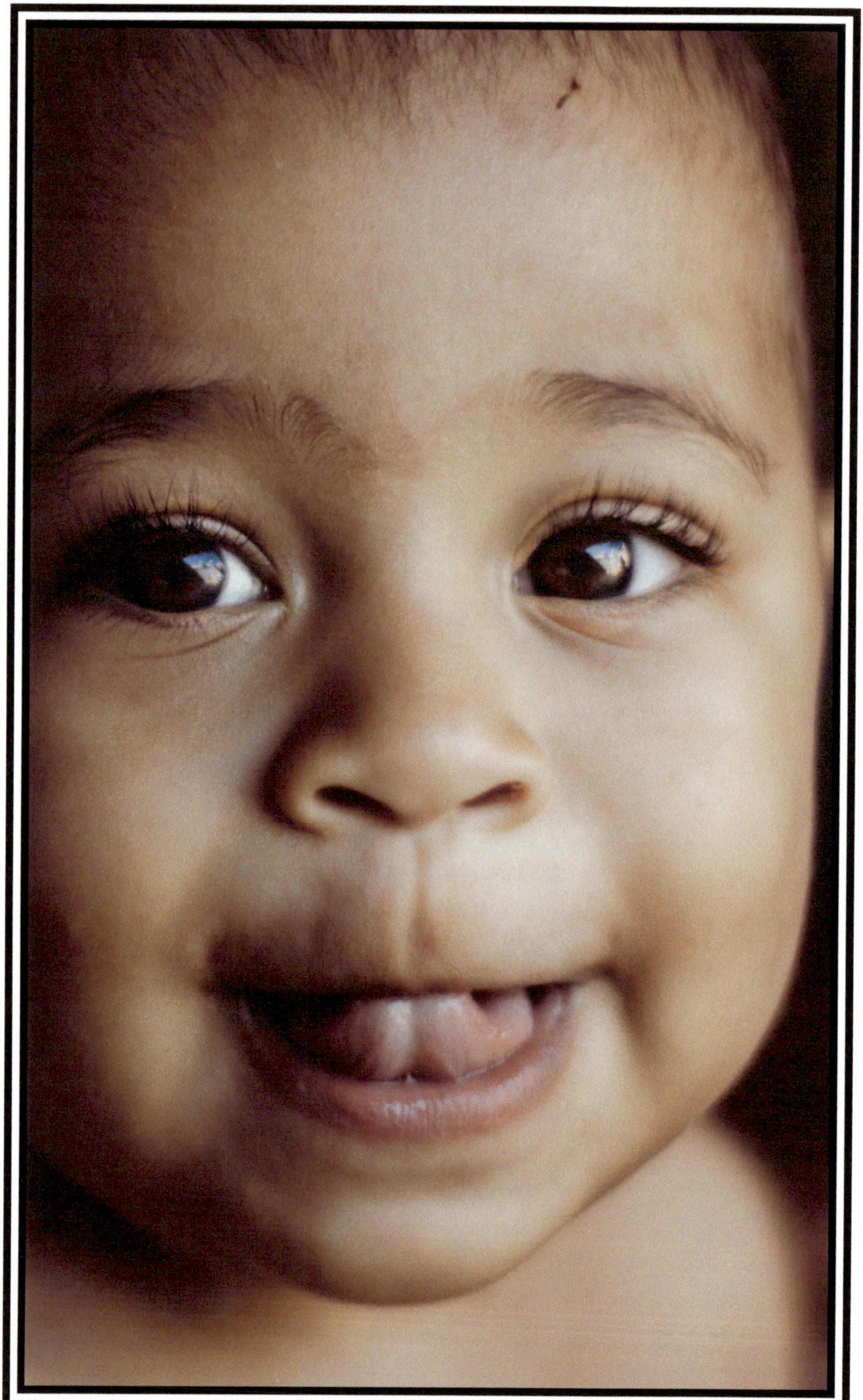

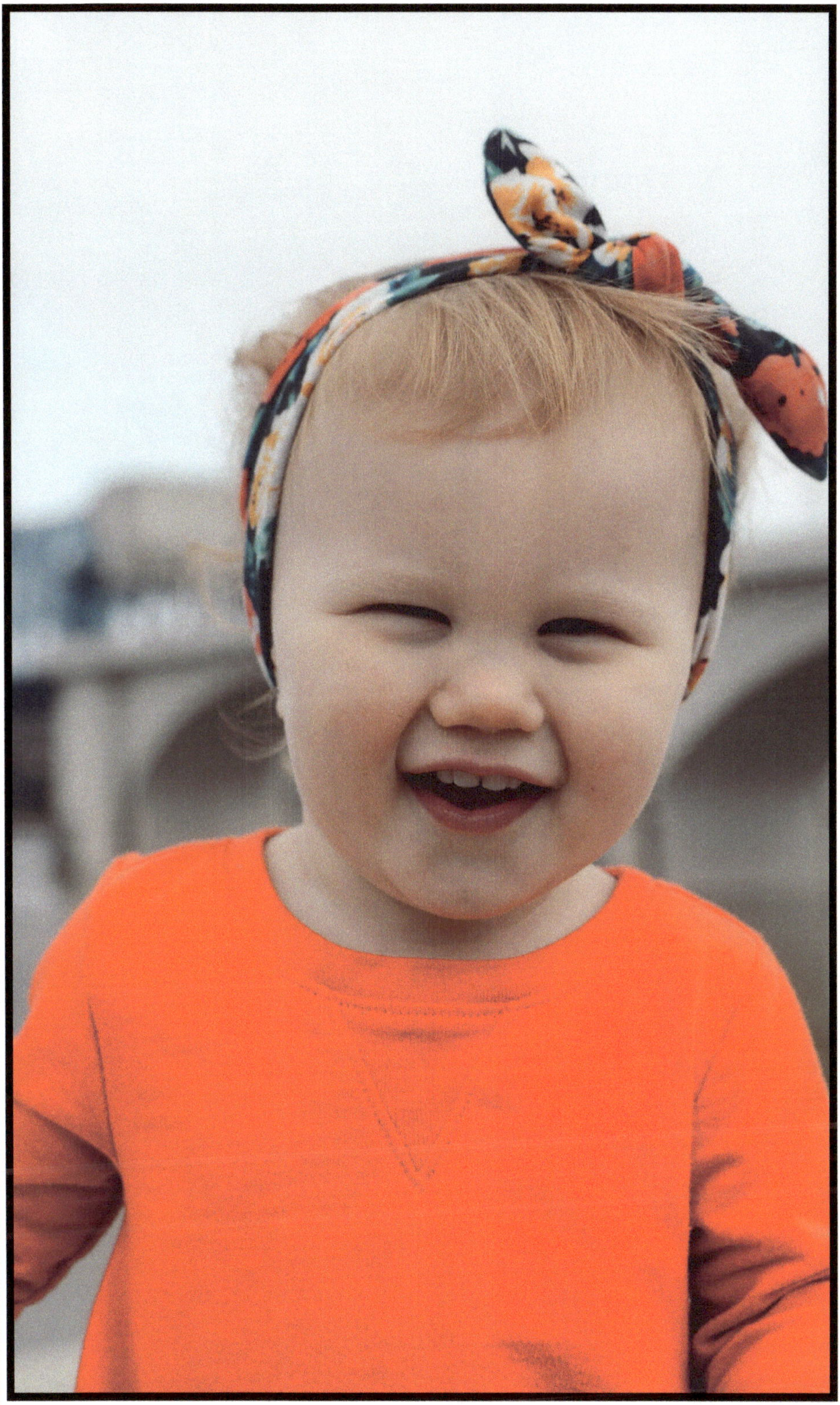

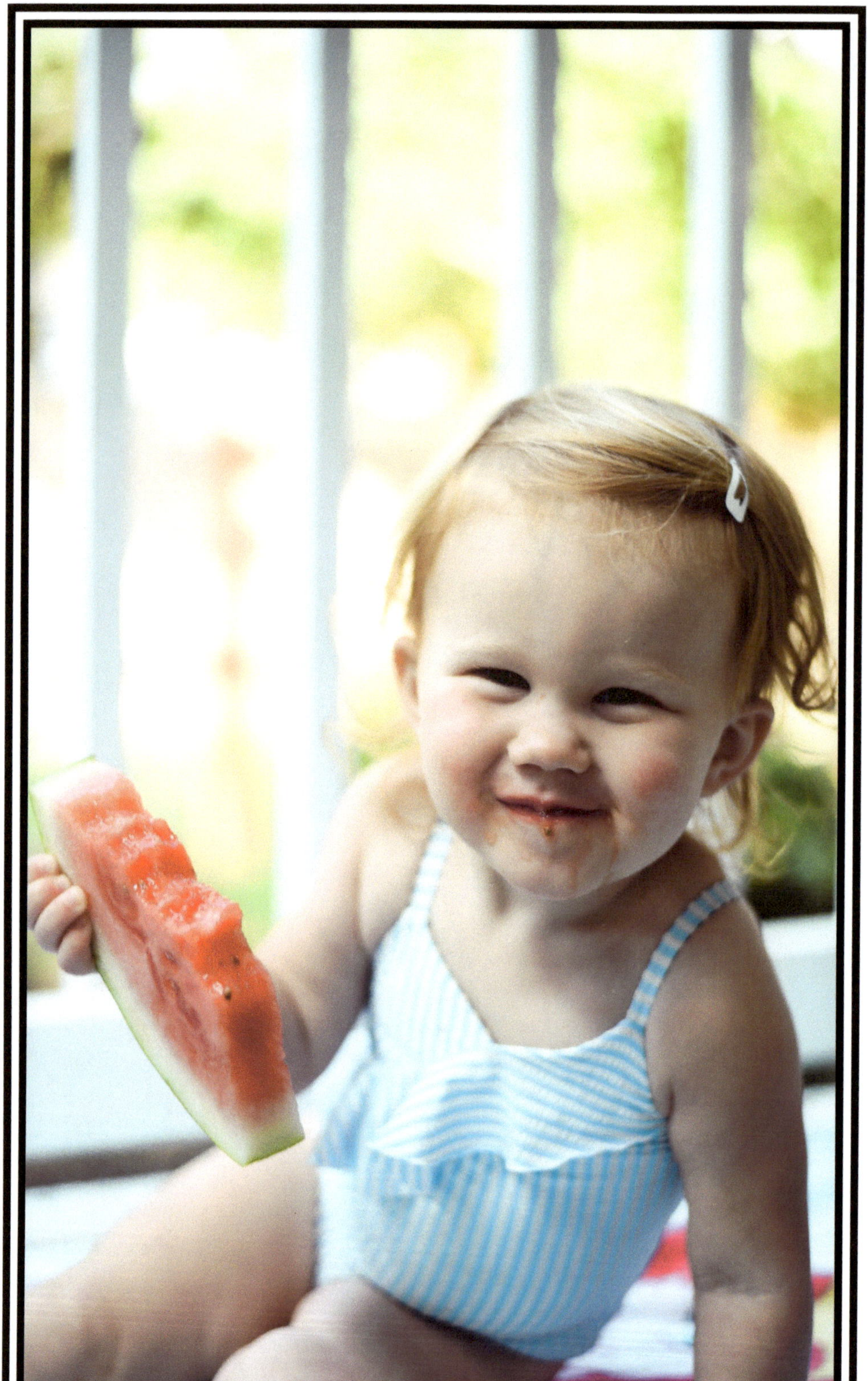

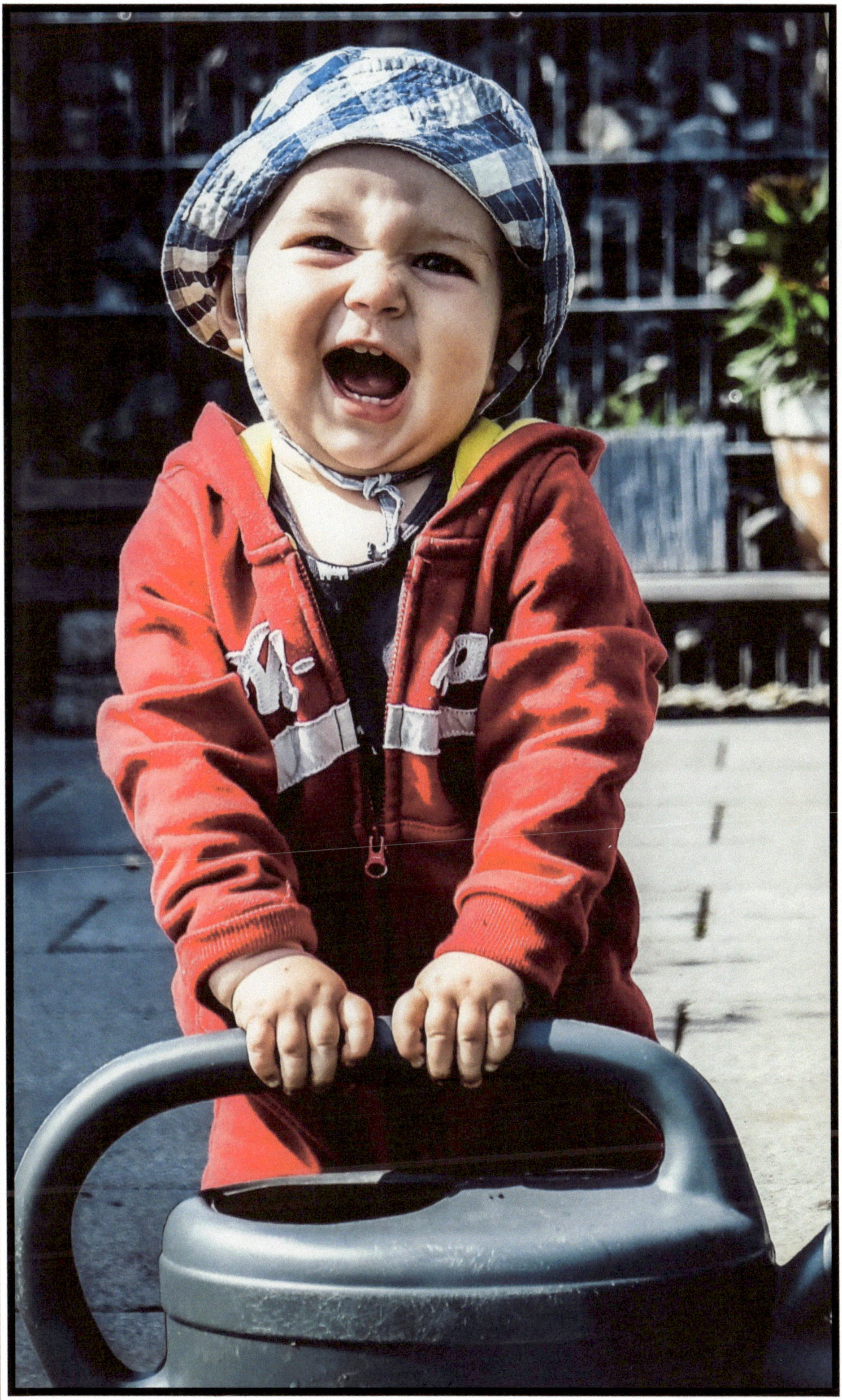

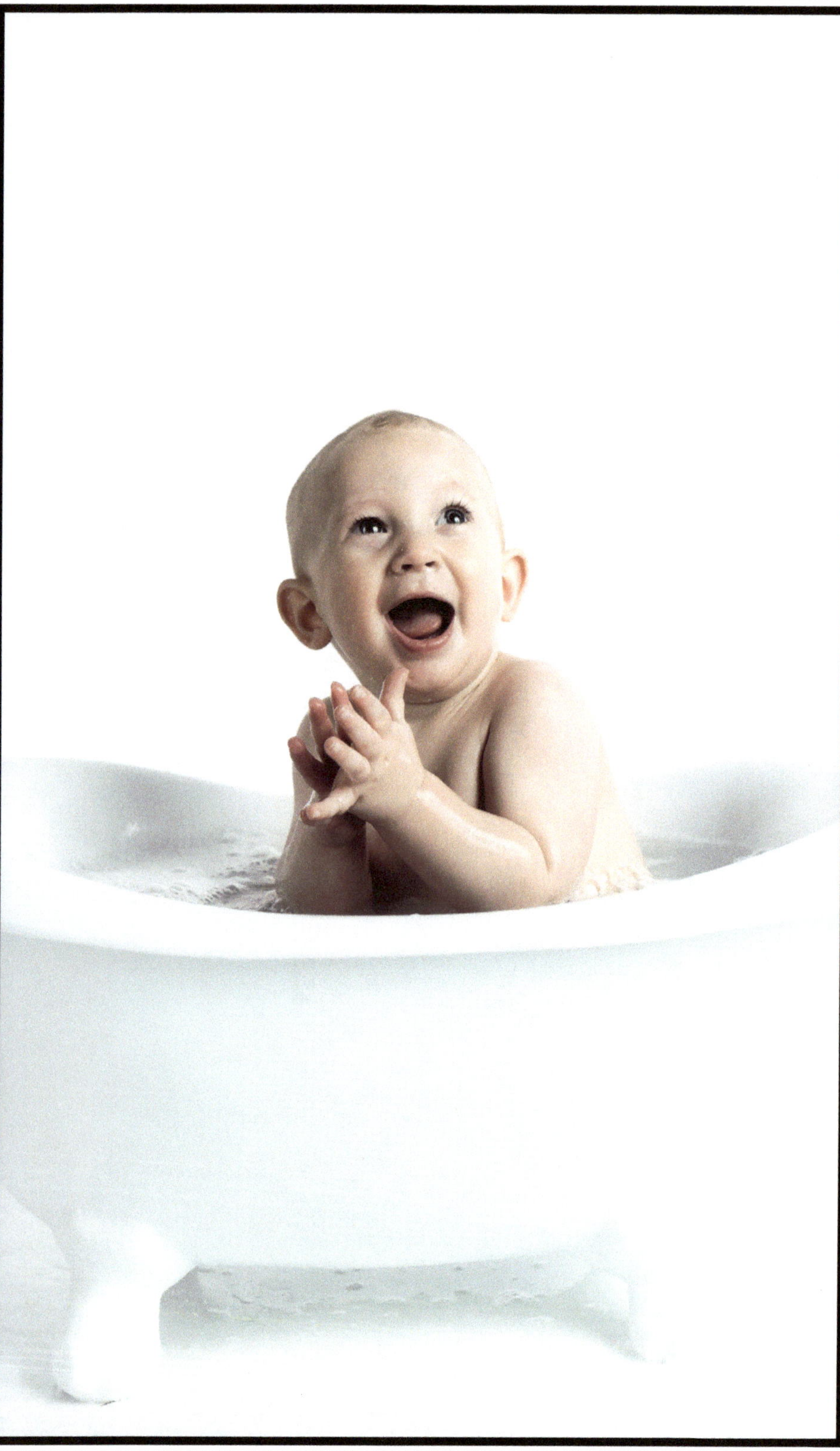

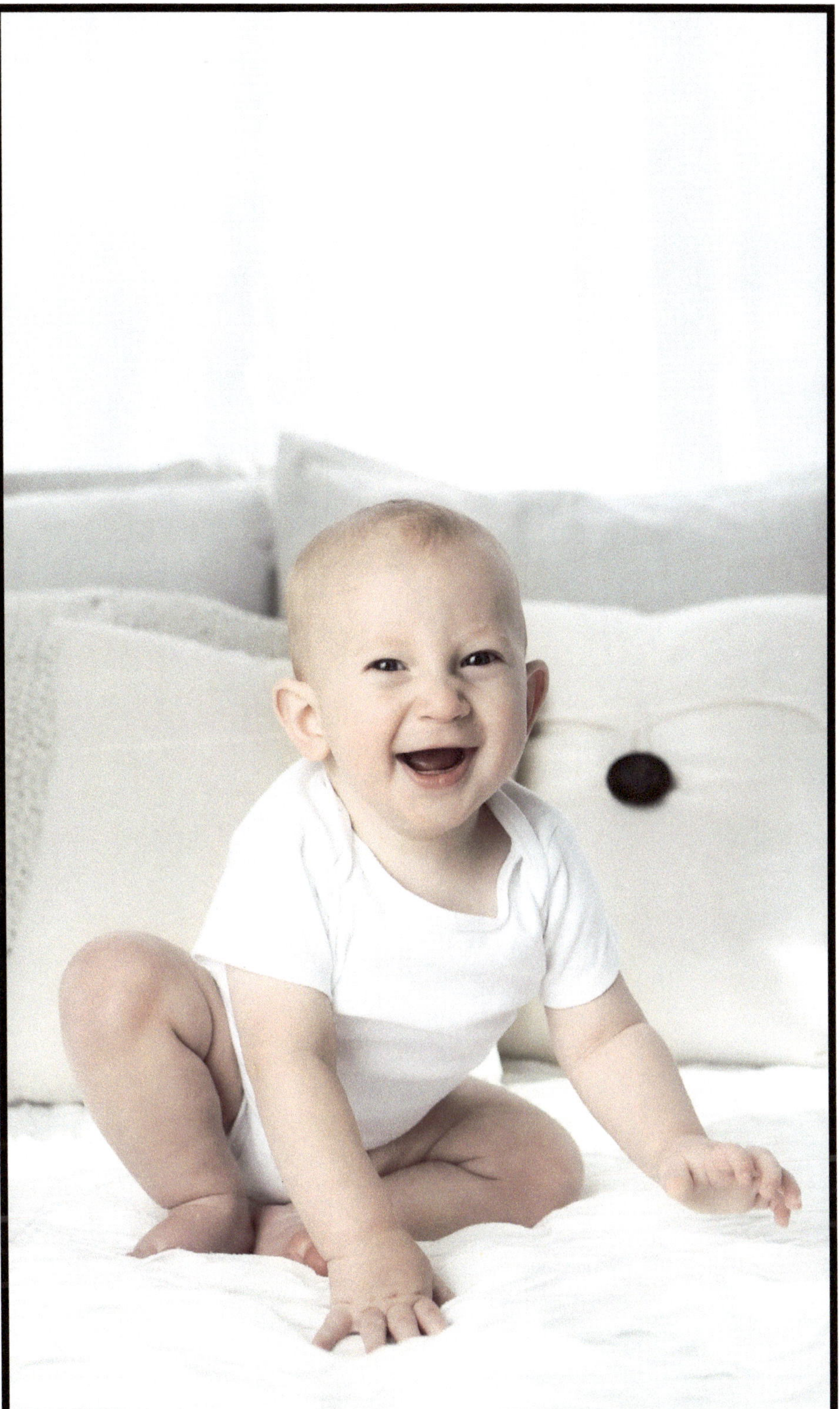

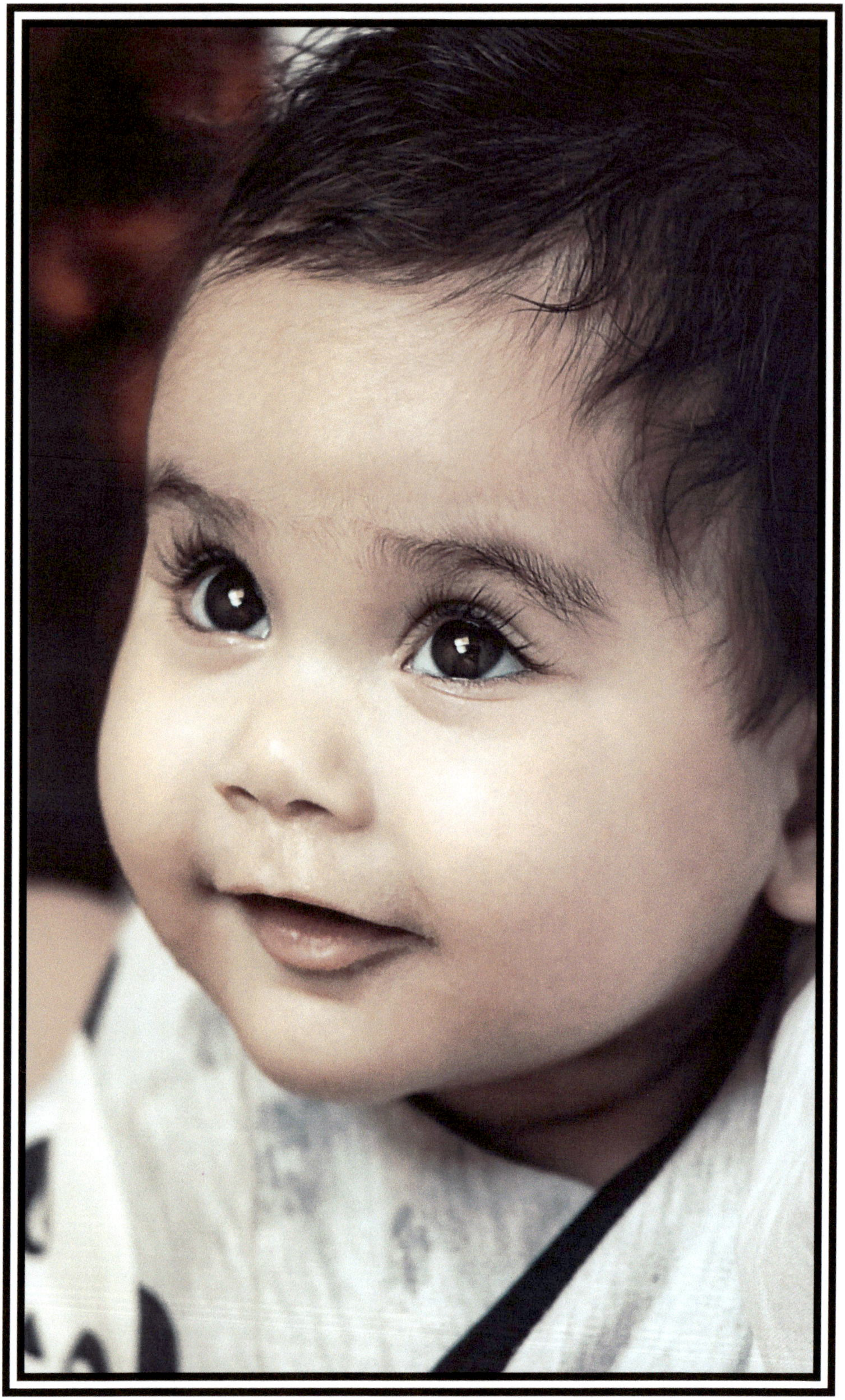

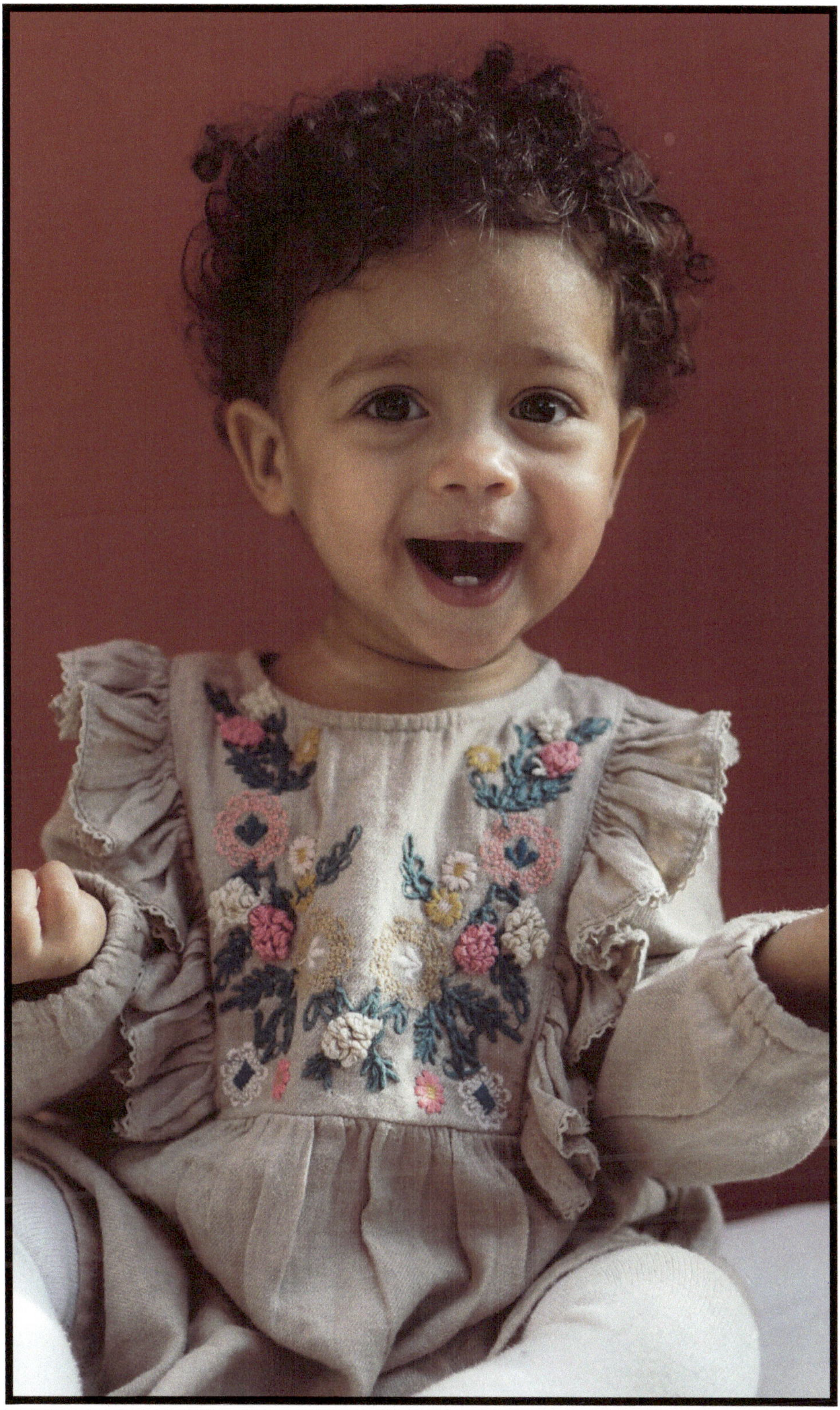

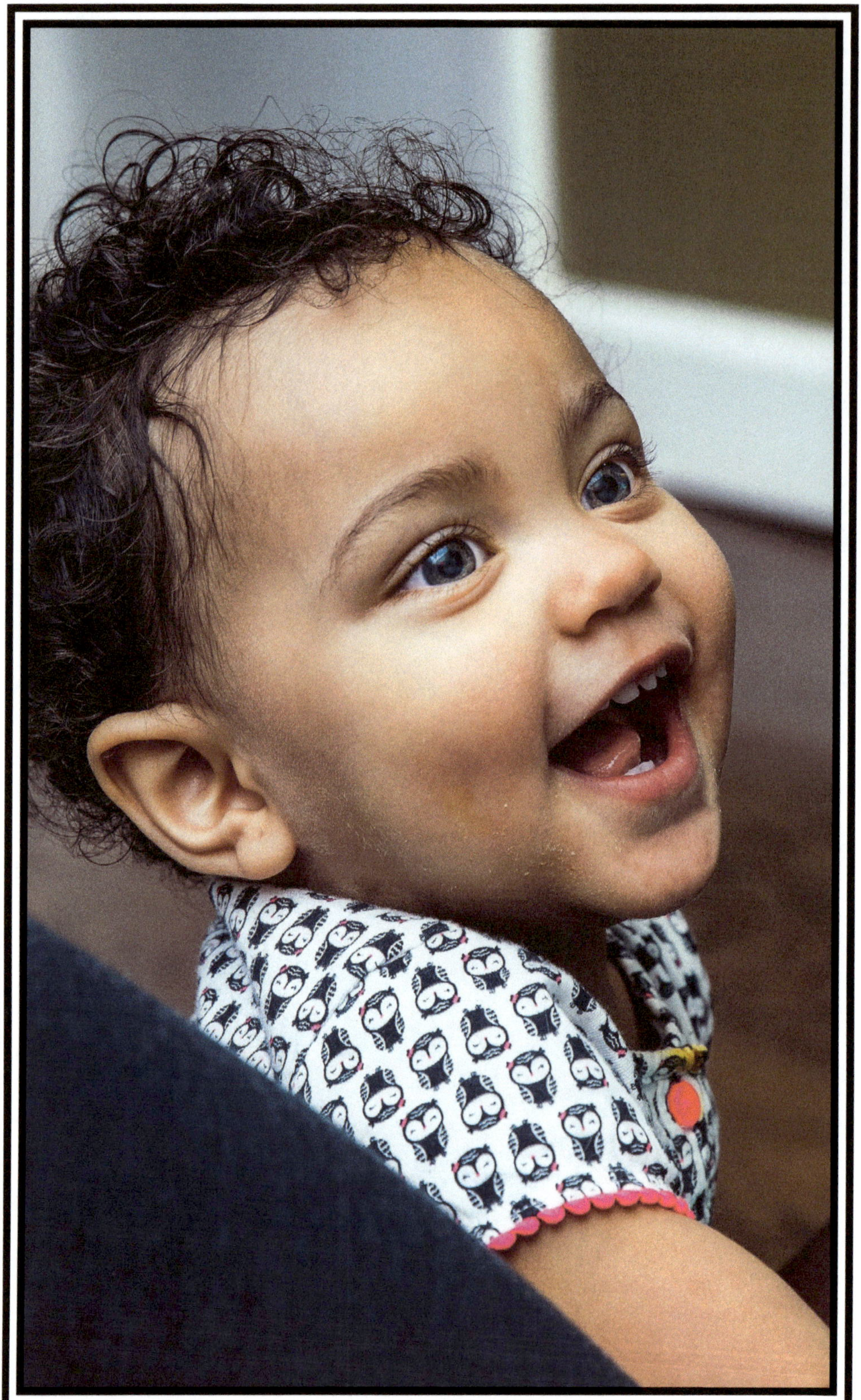

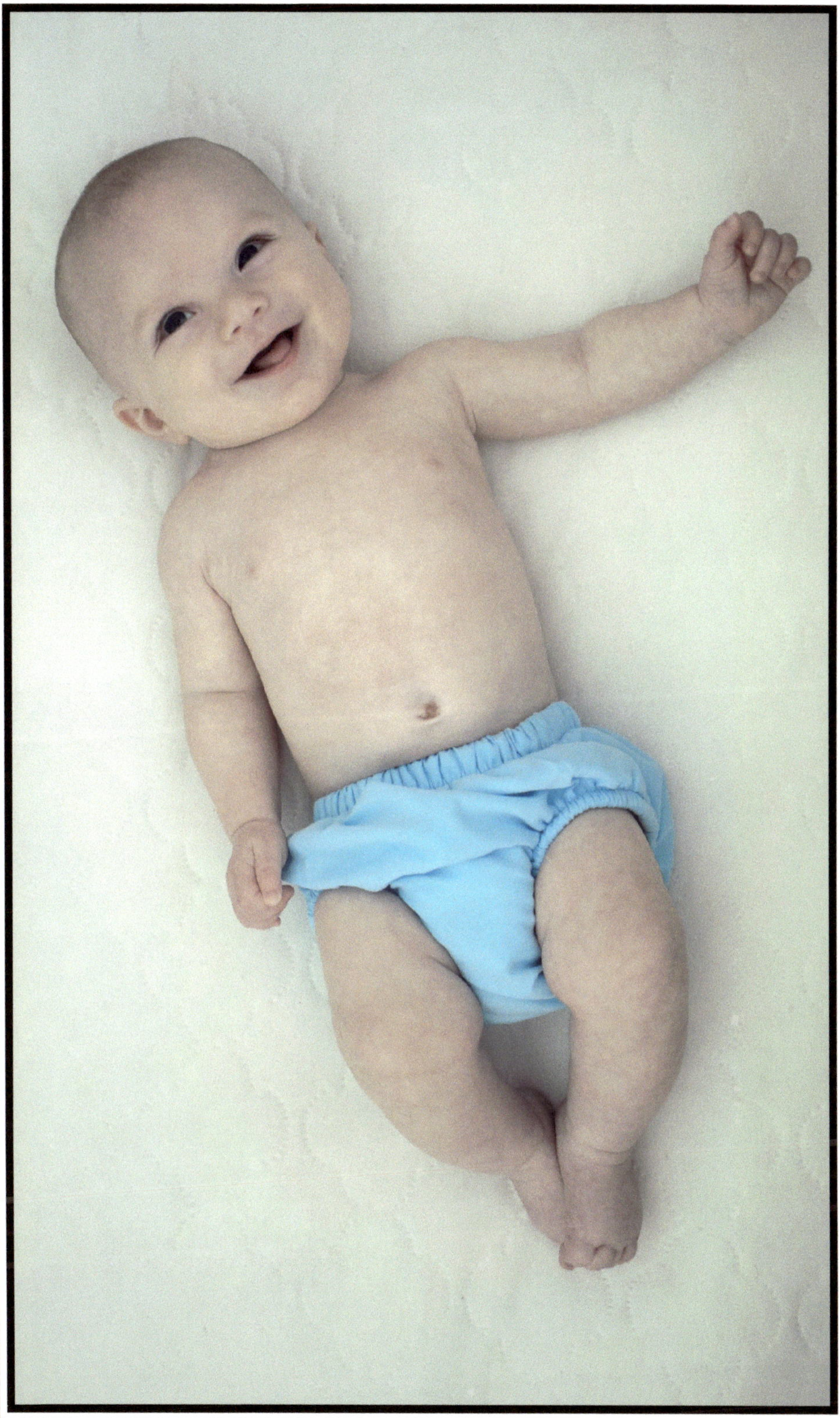

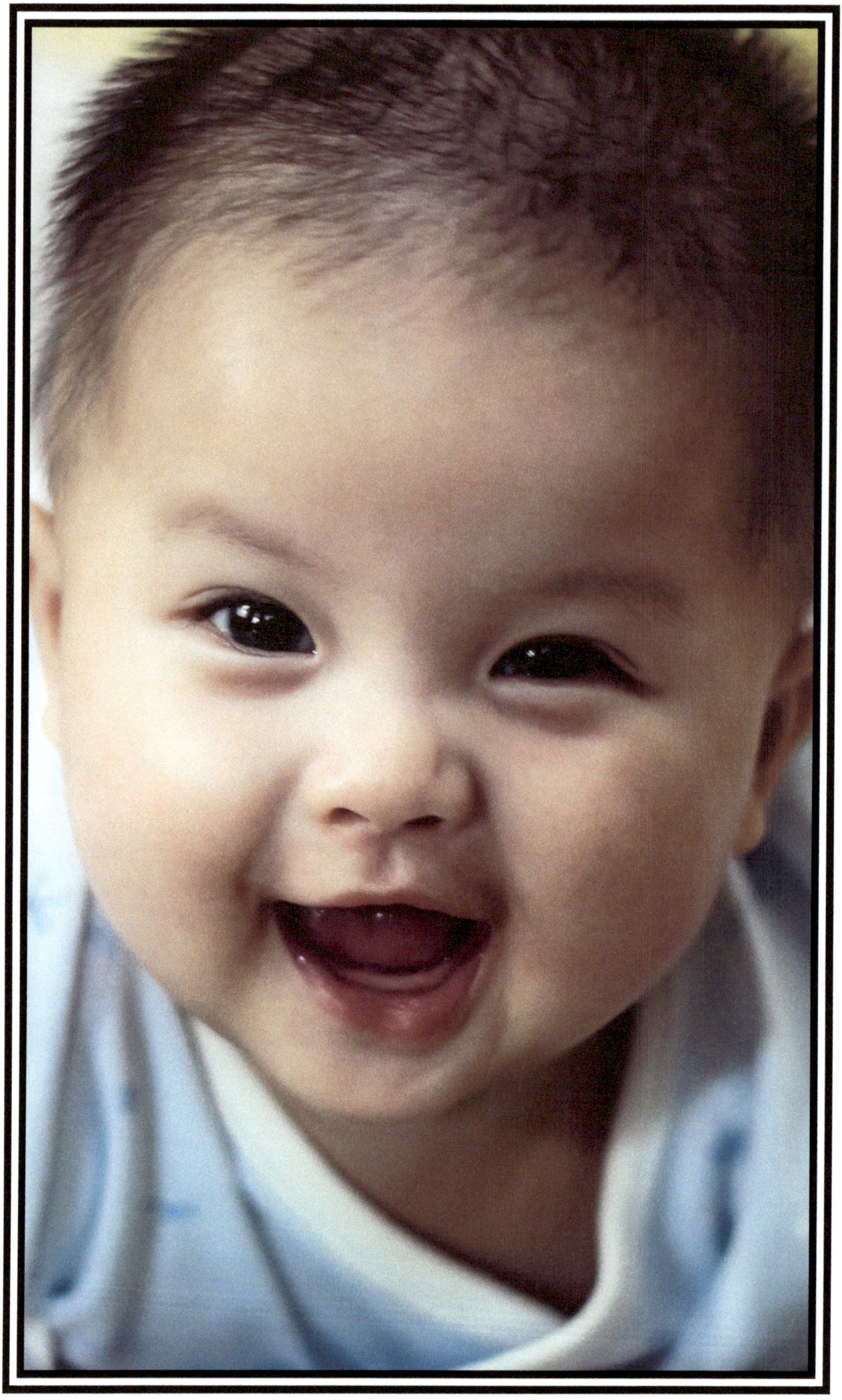

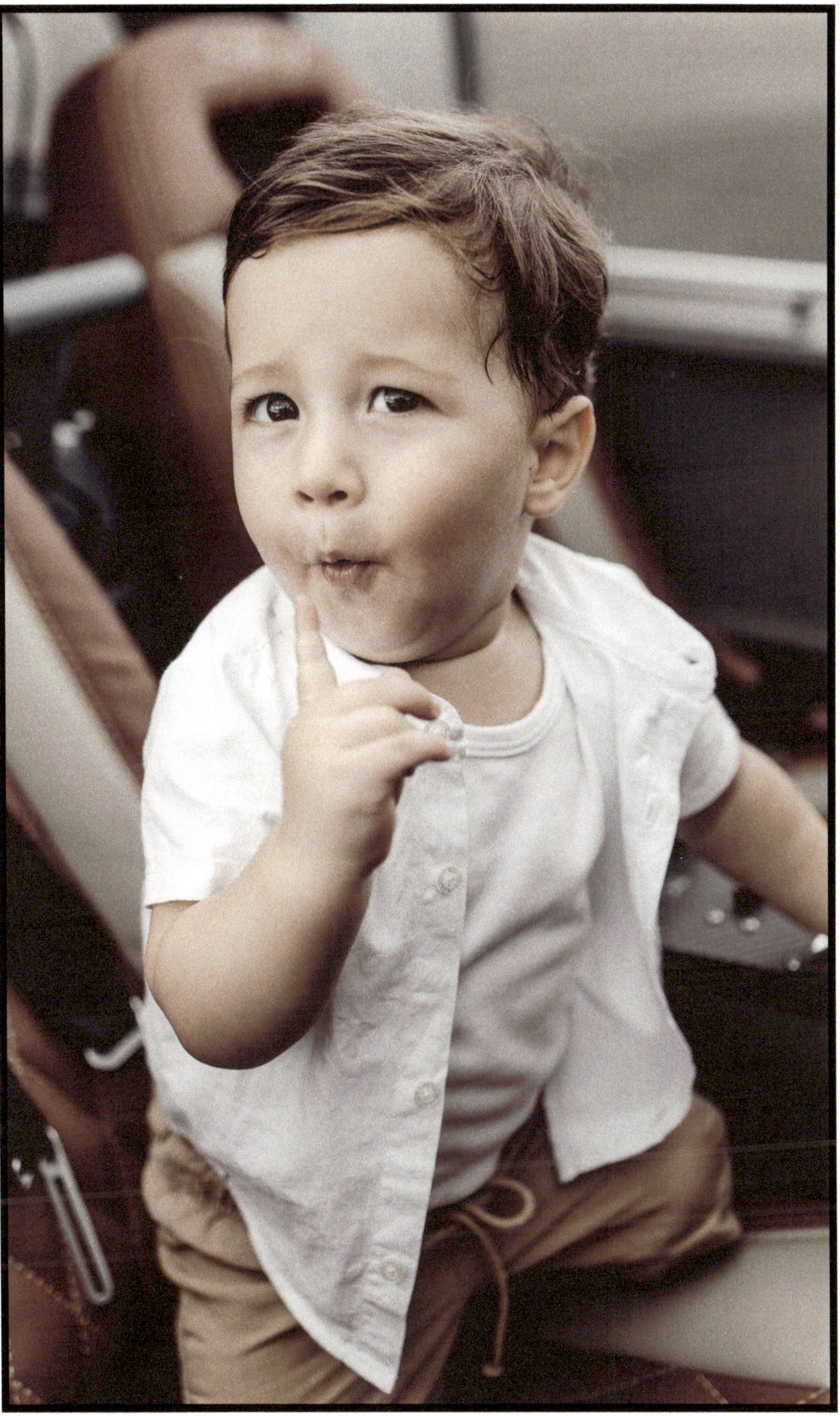

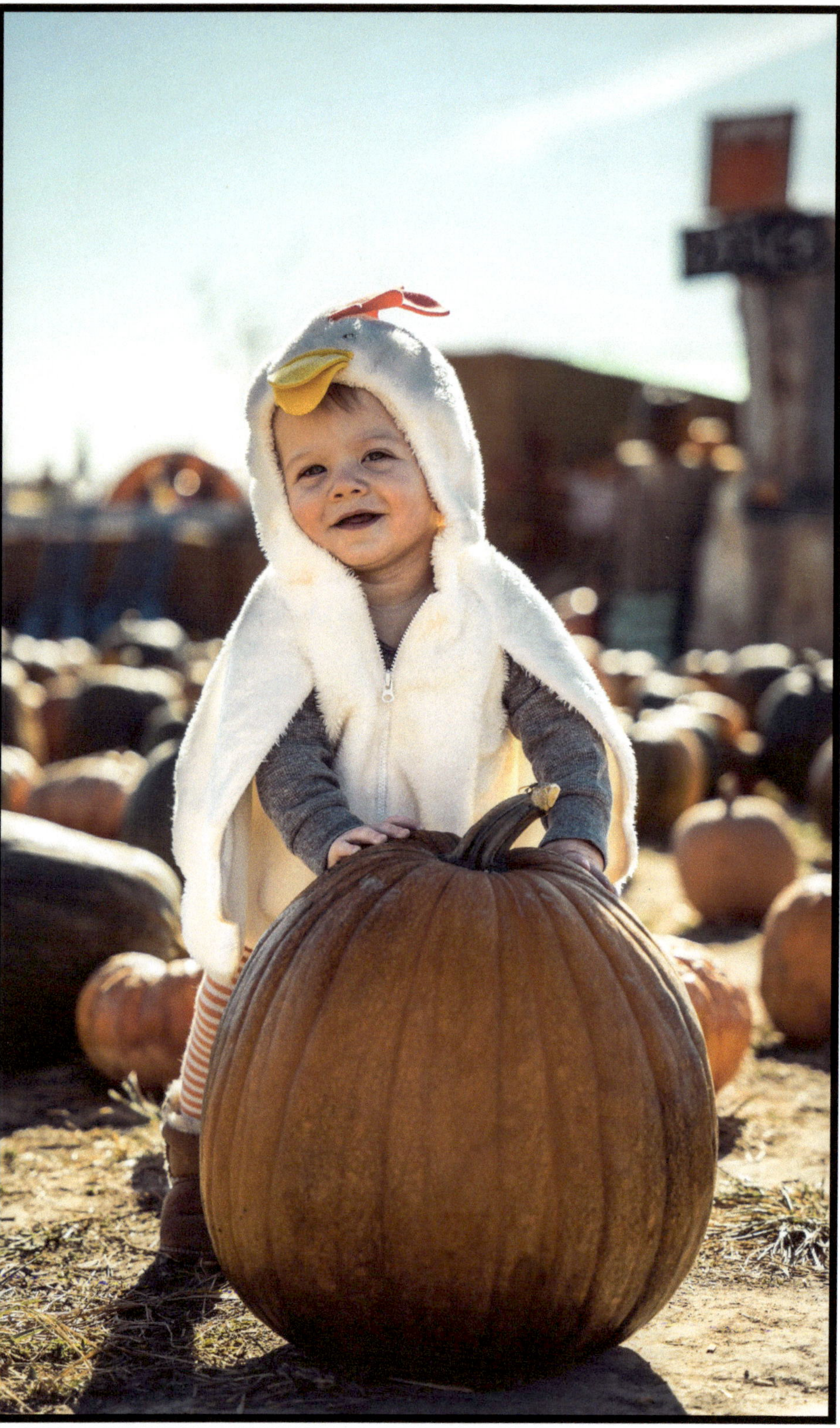

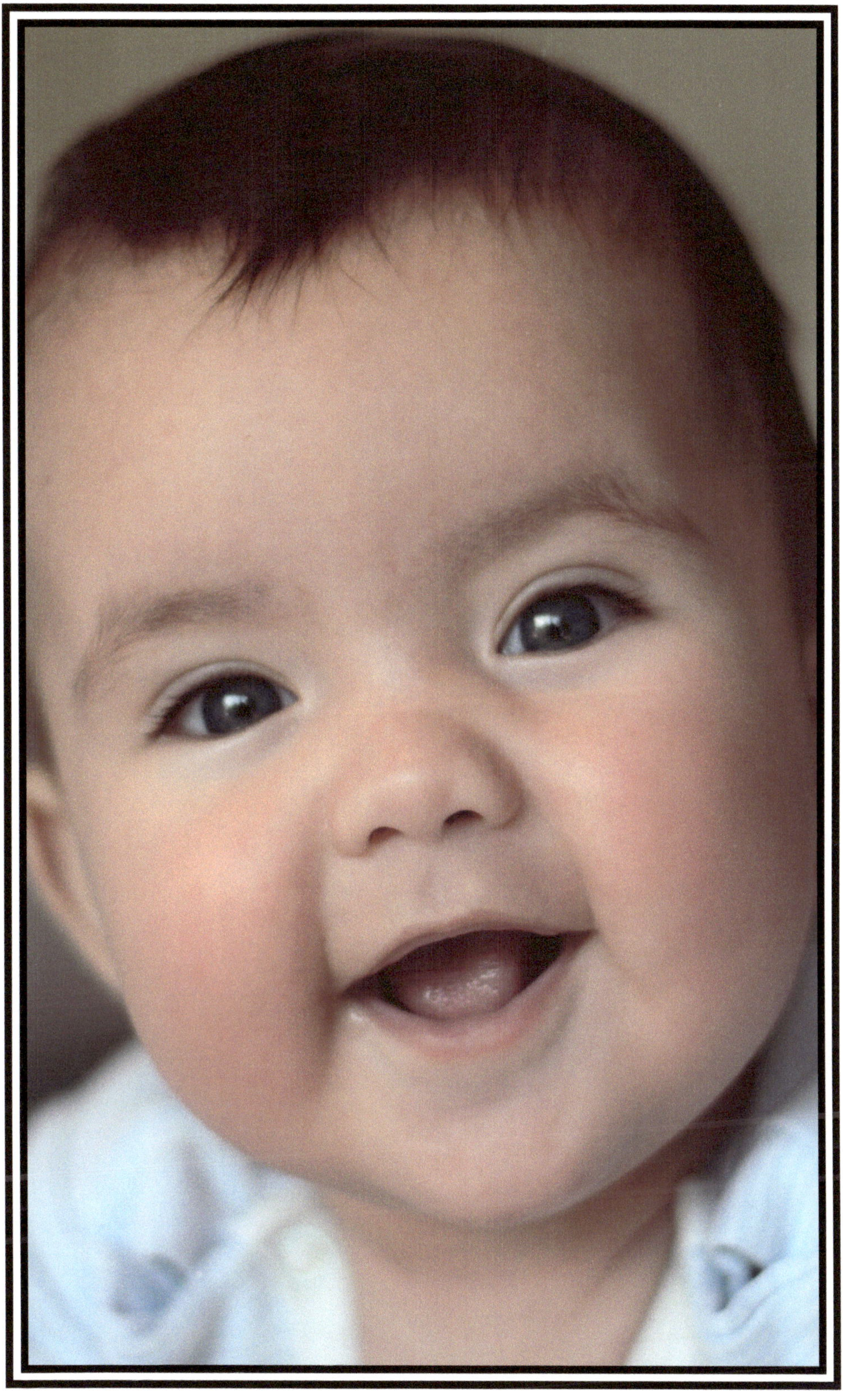

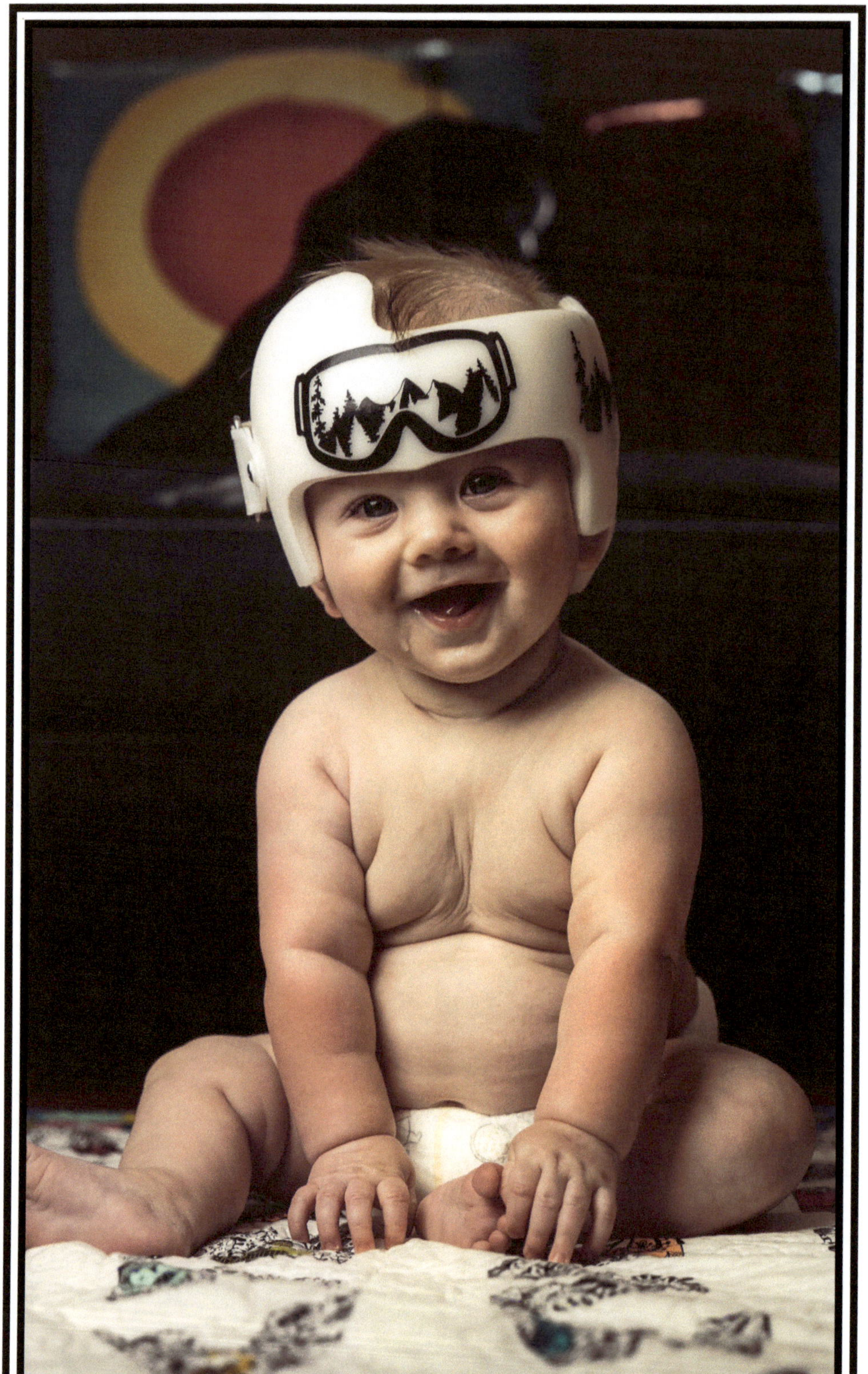

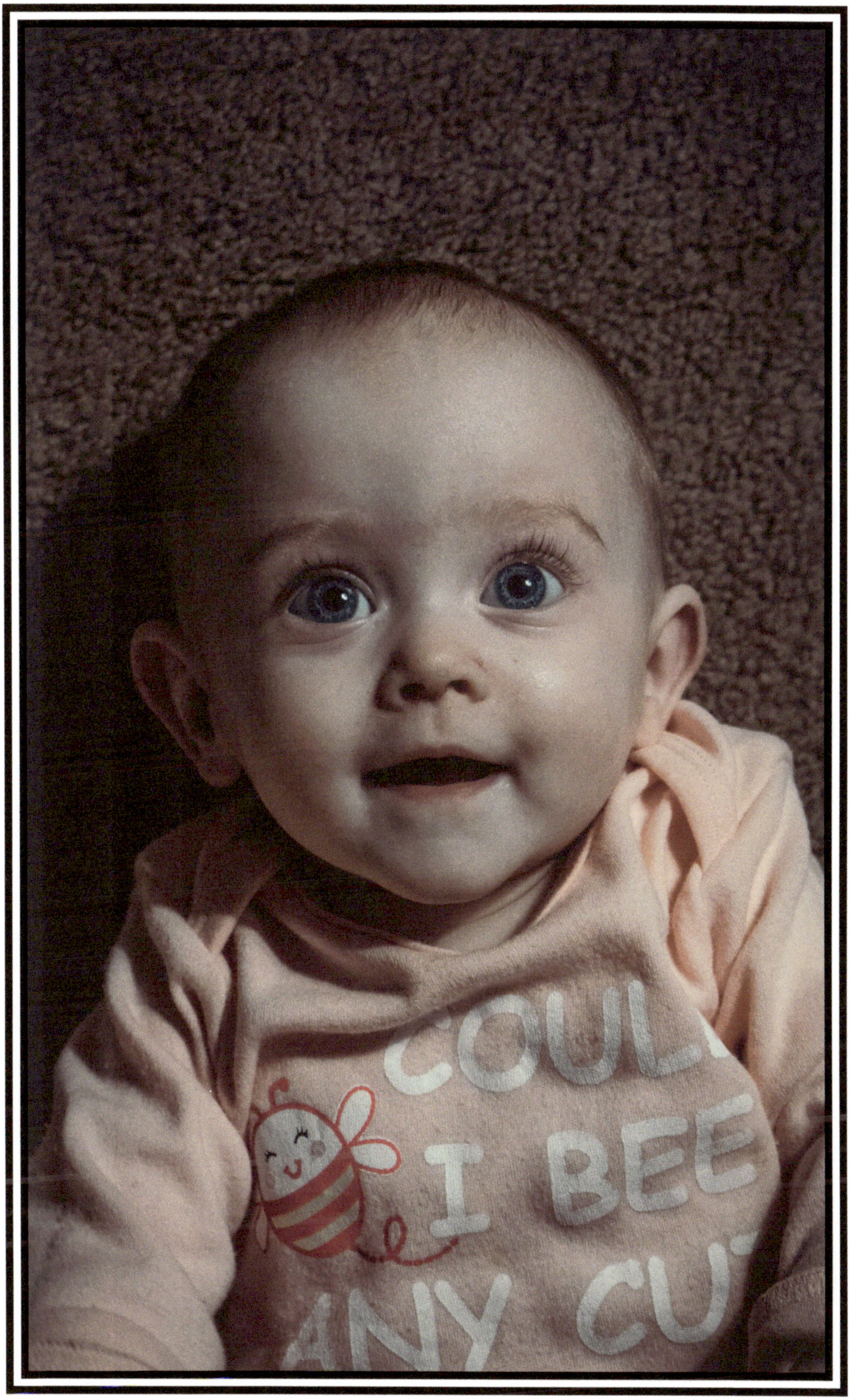

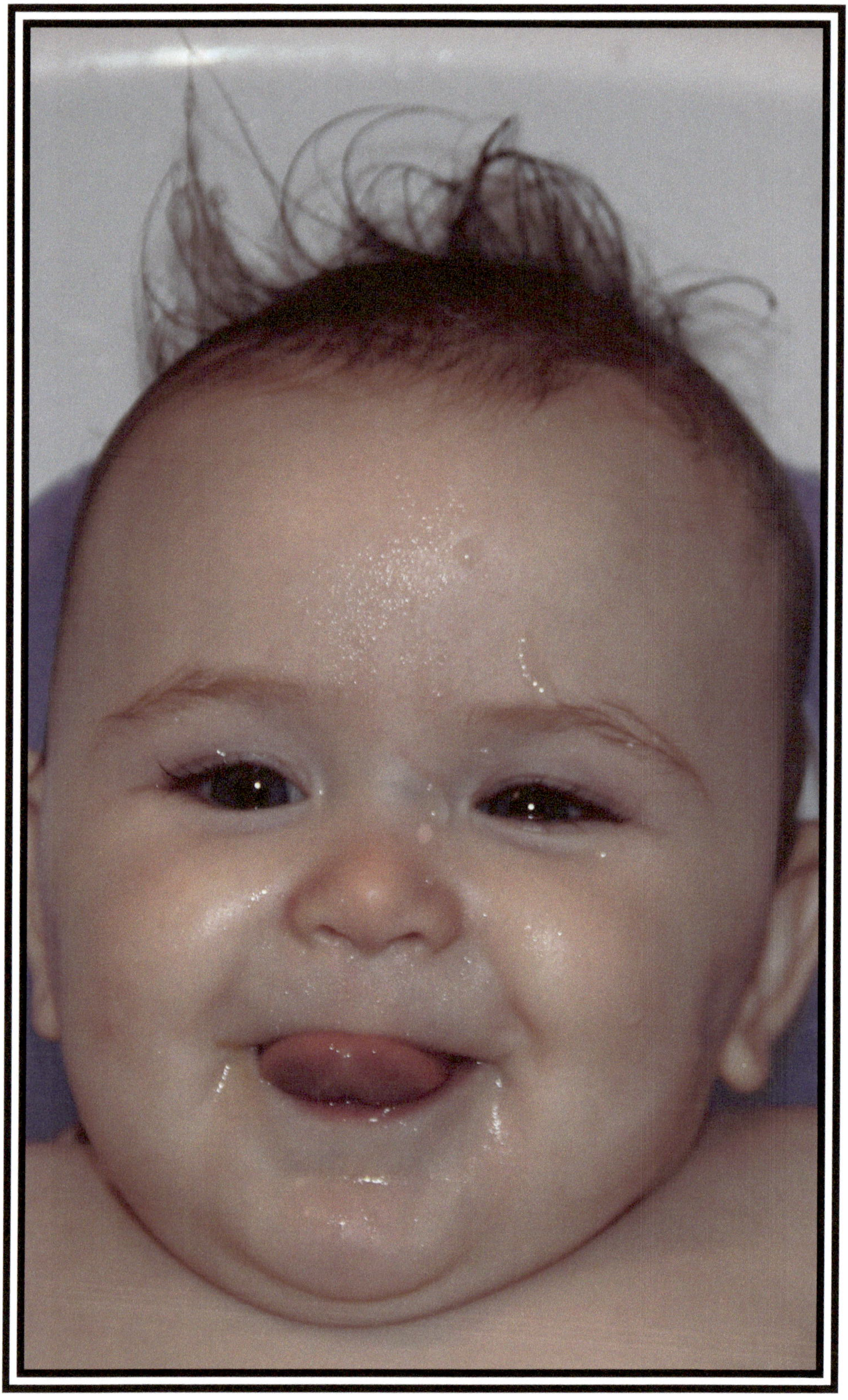

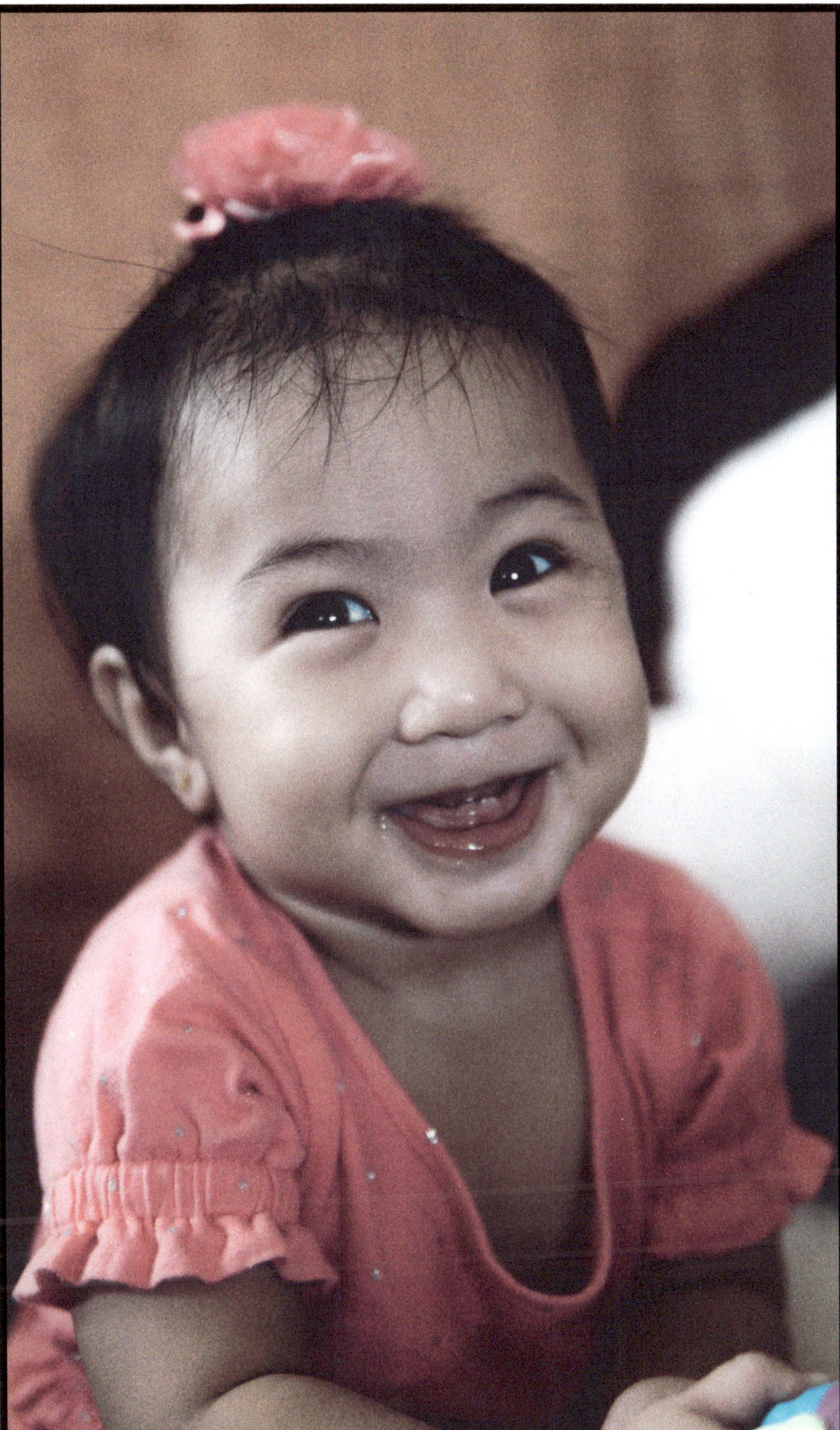

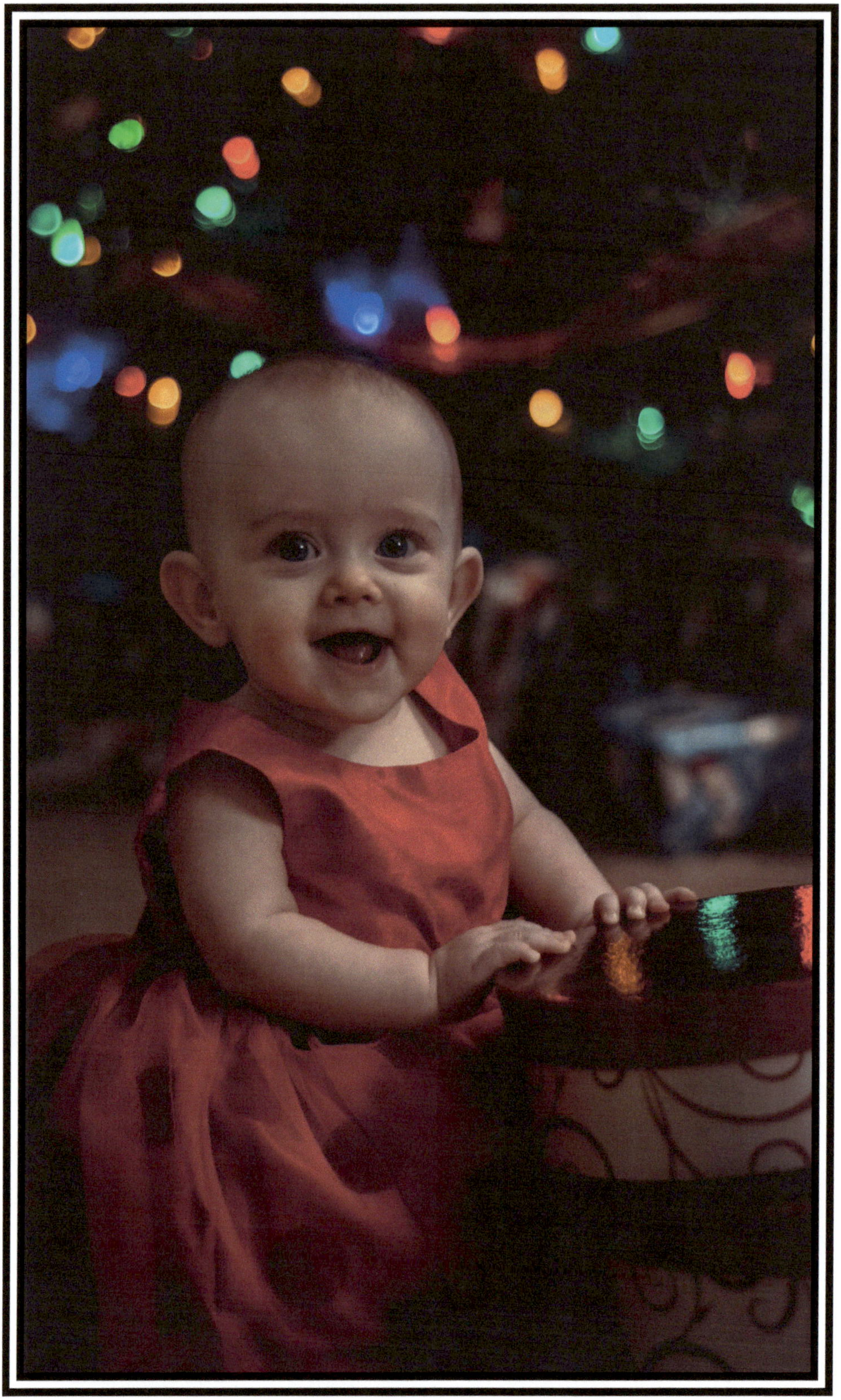

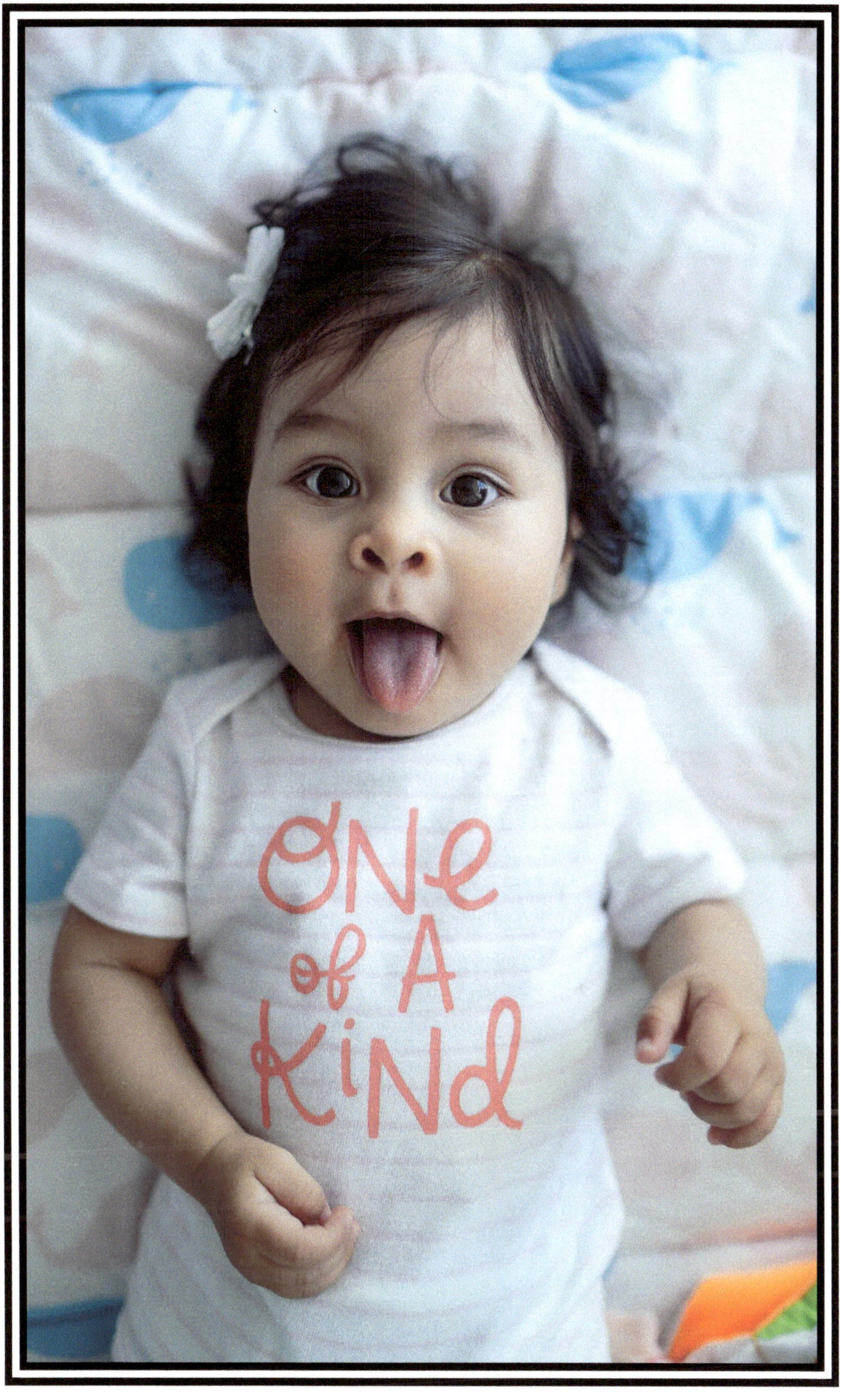
One of A Kind

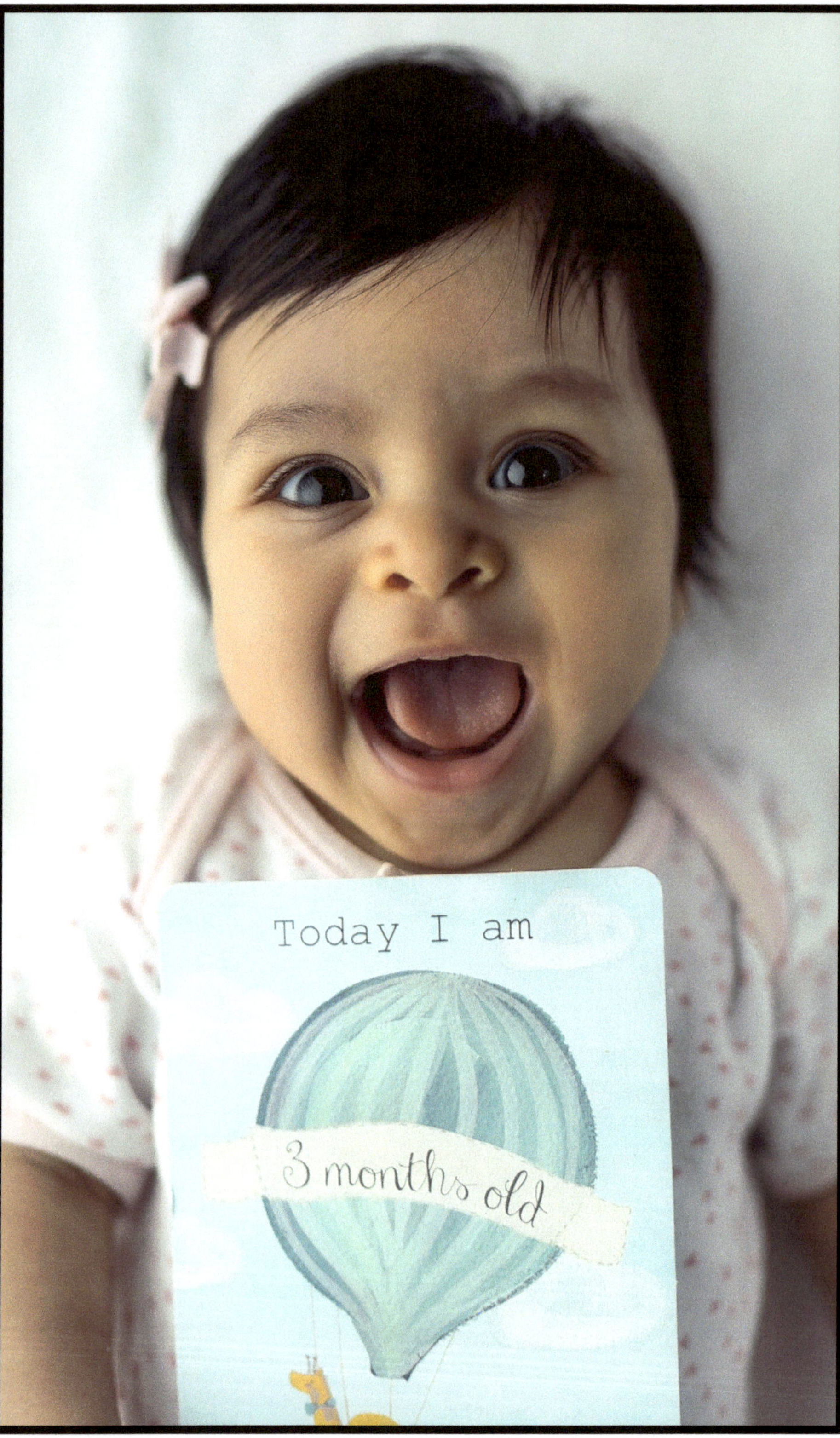
Today I am
3 months old

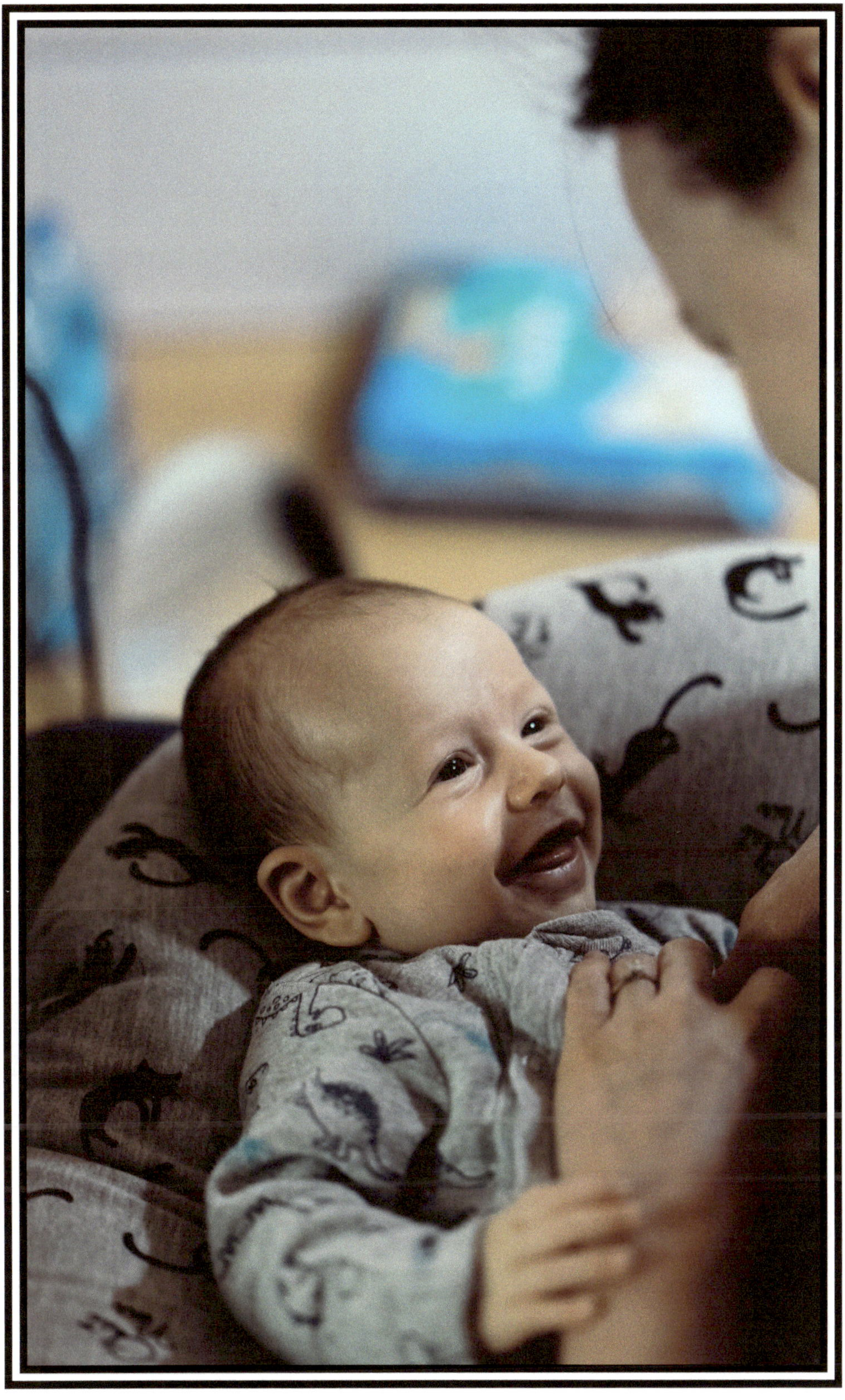

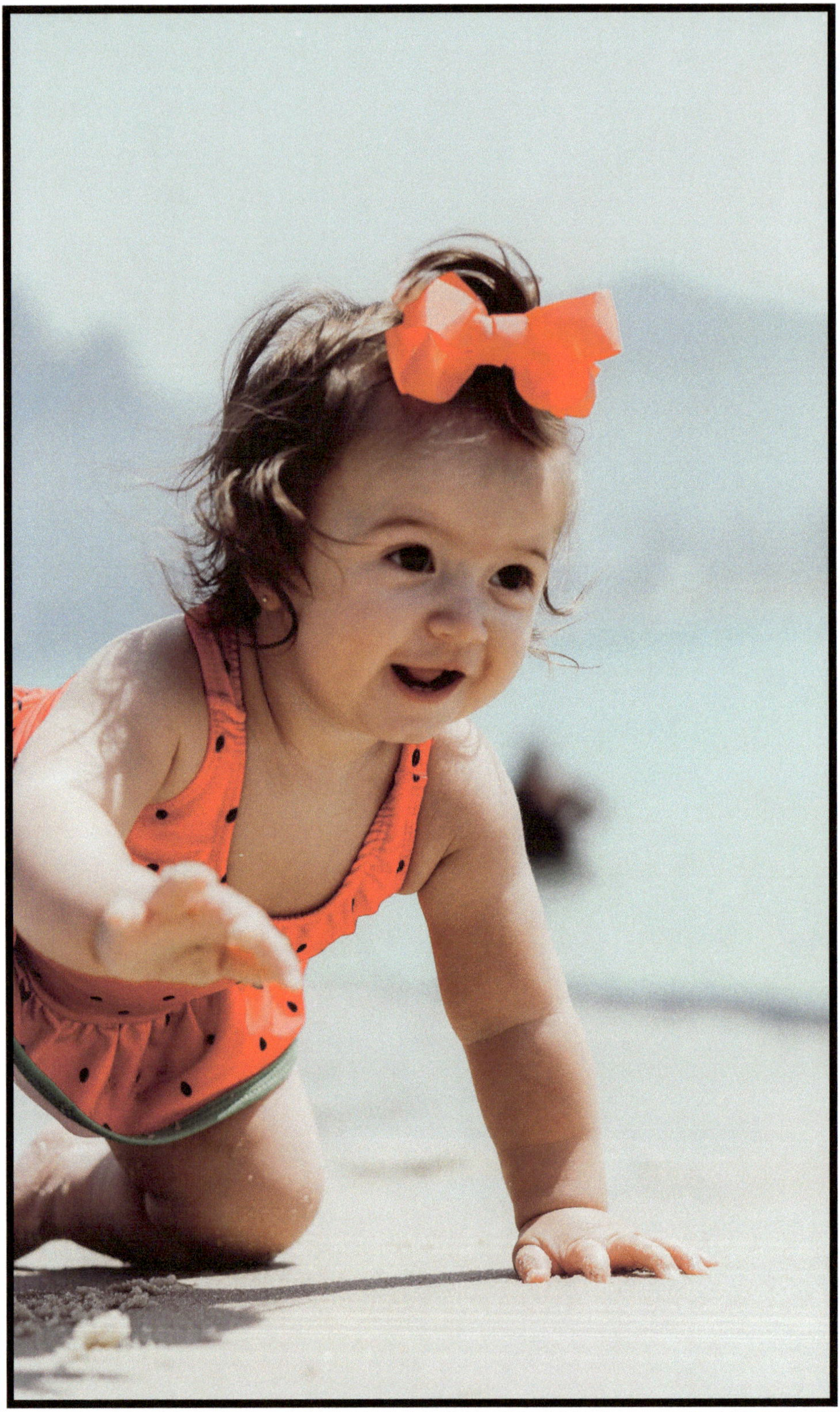

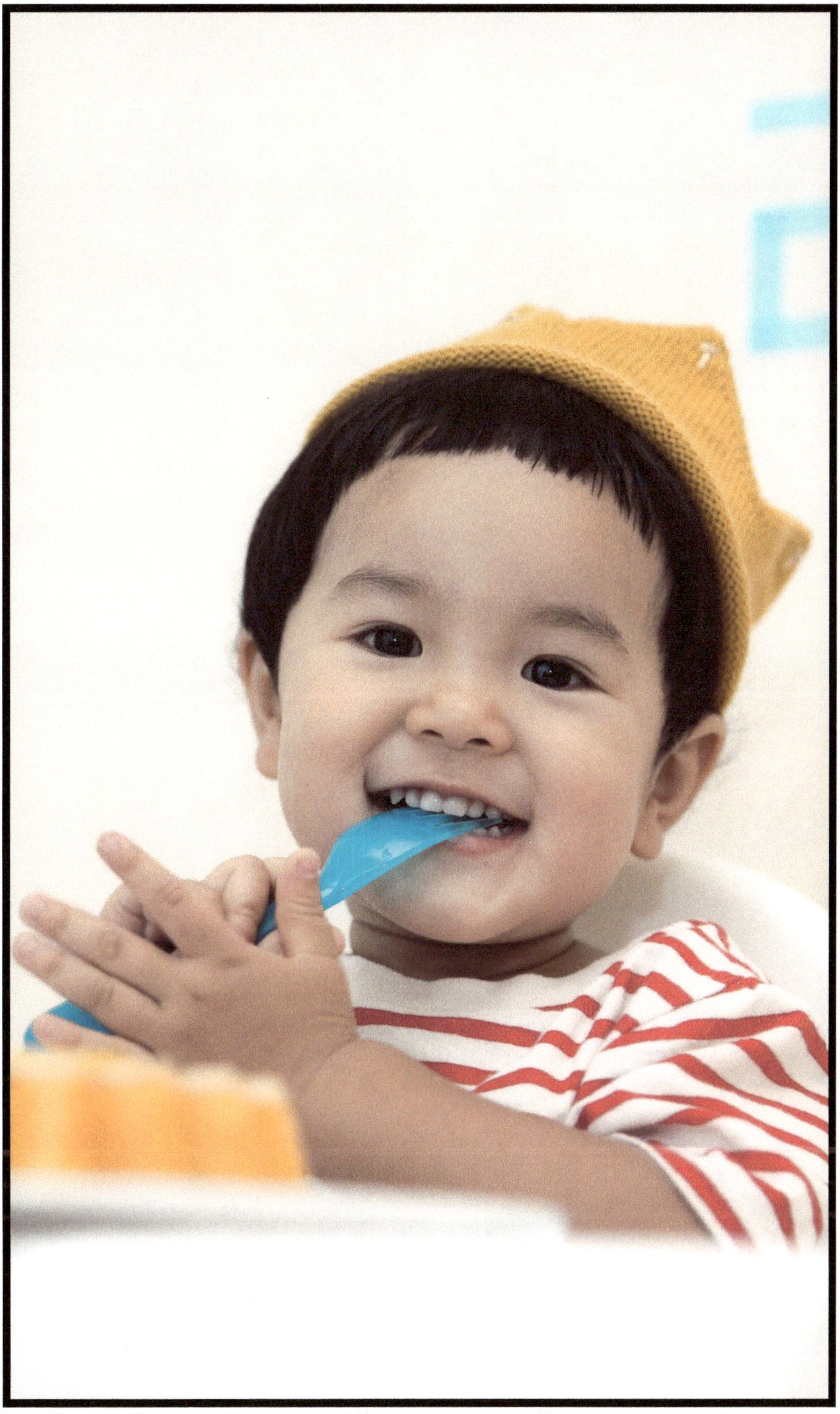

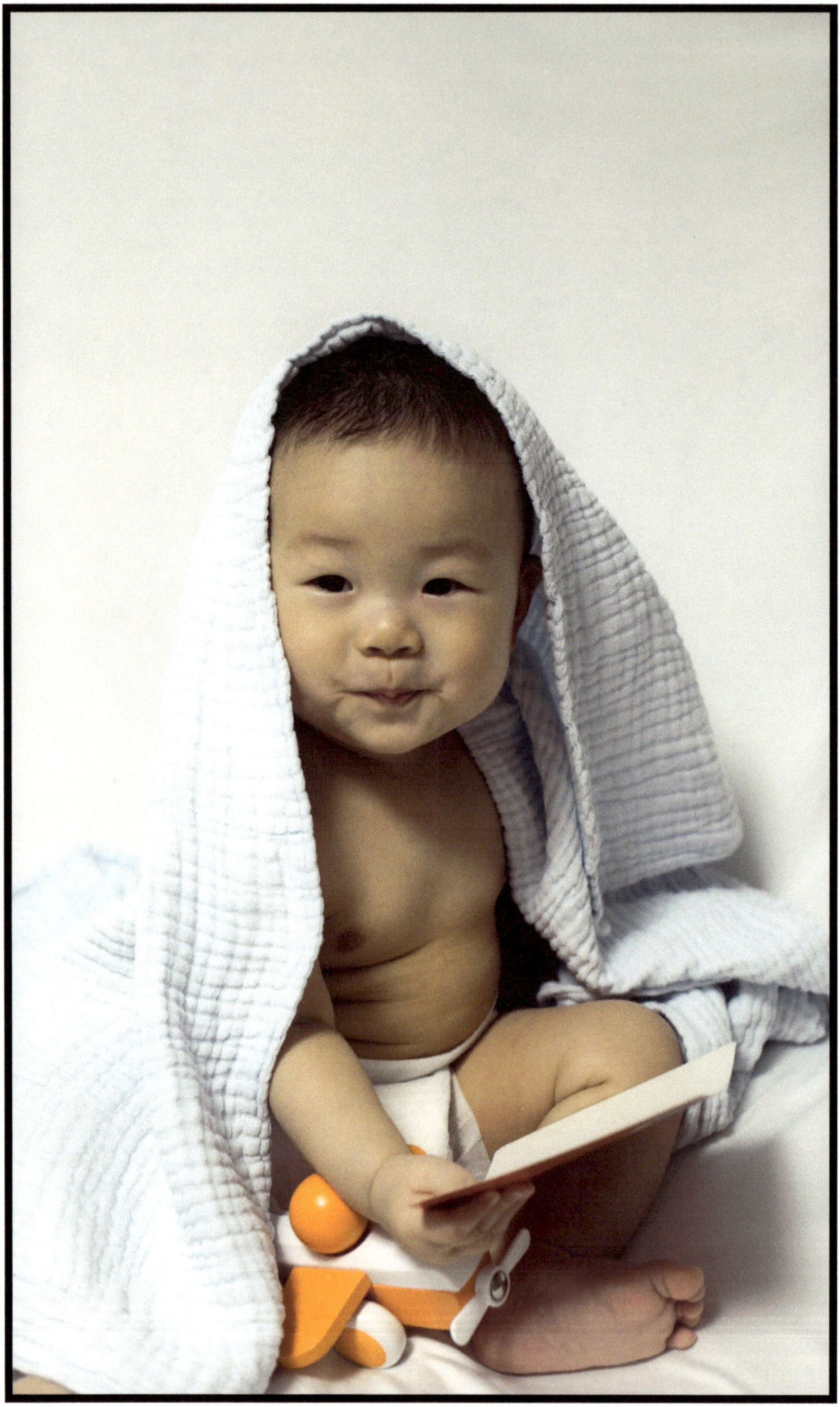

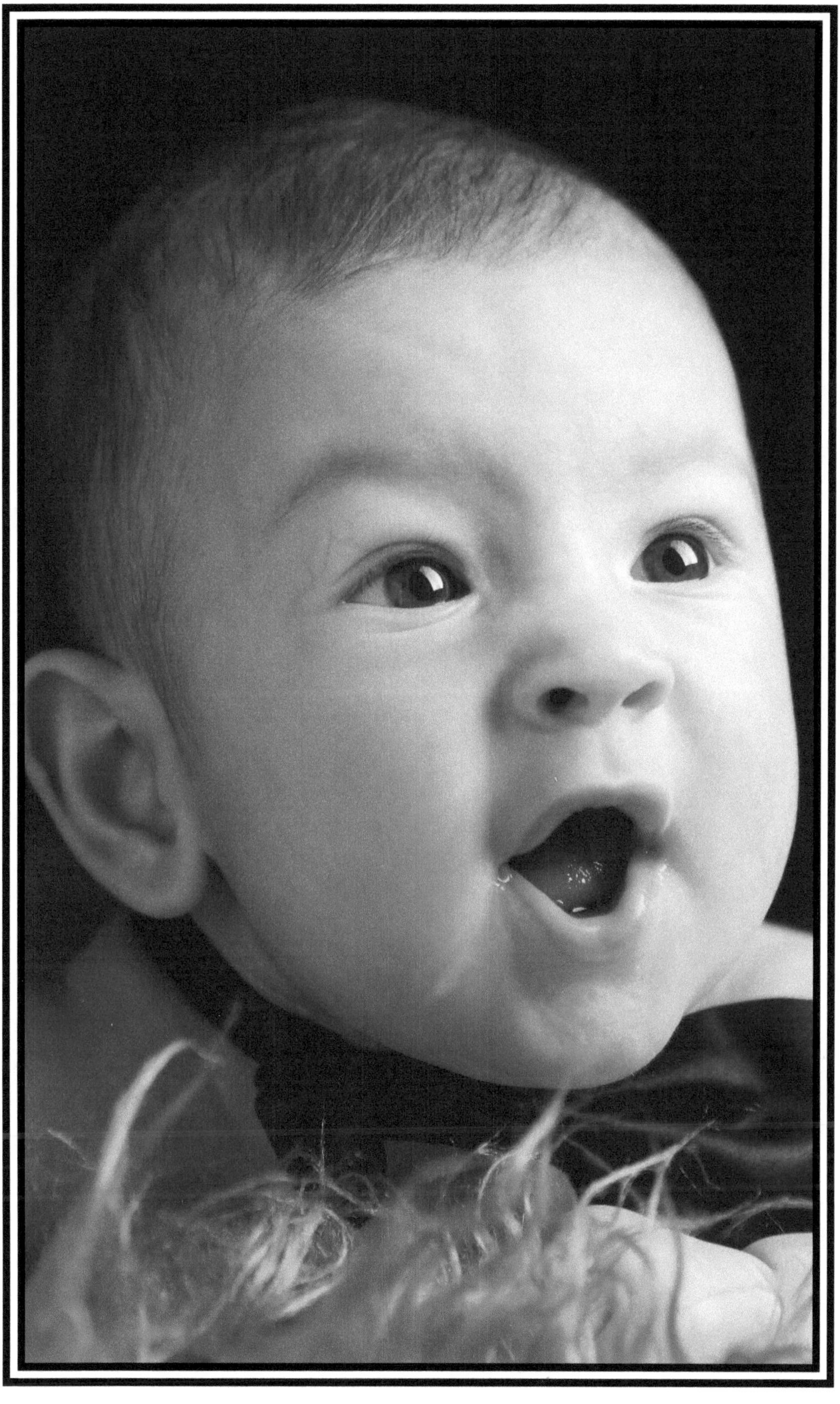

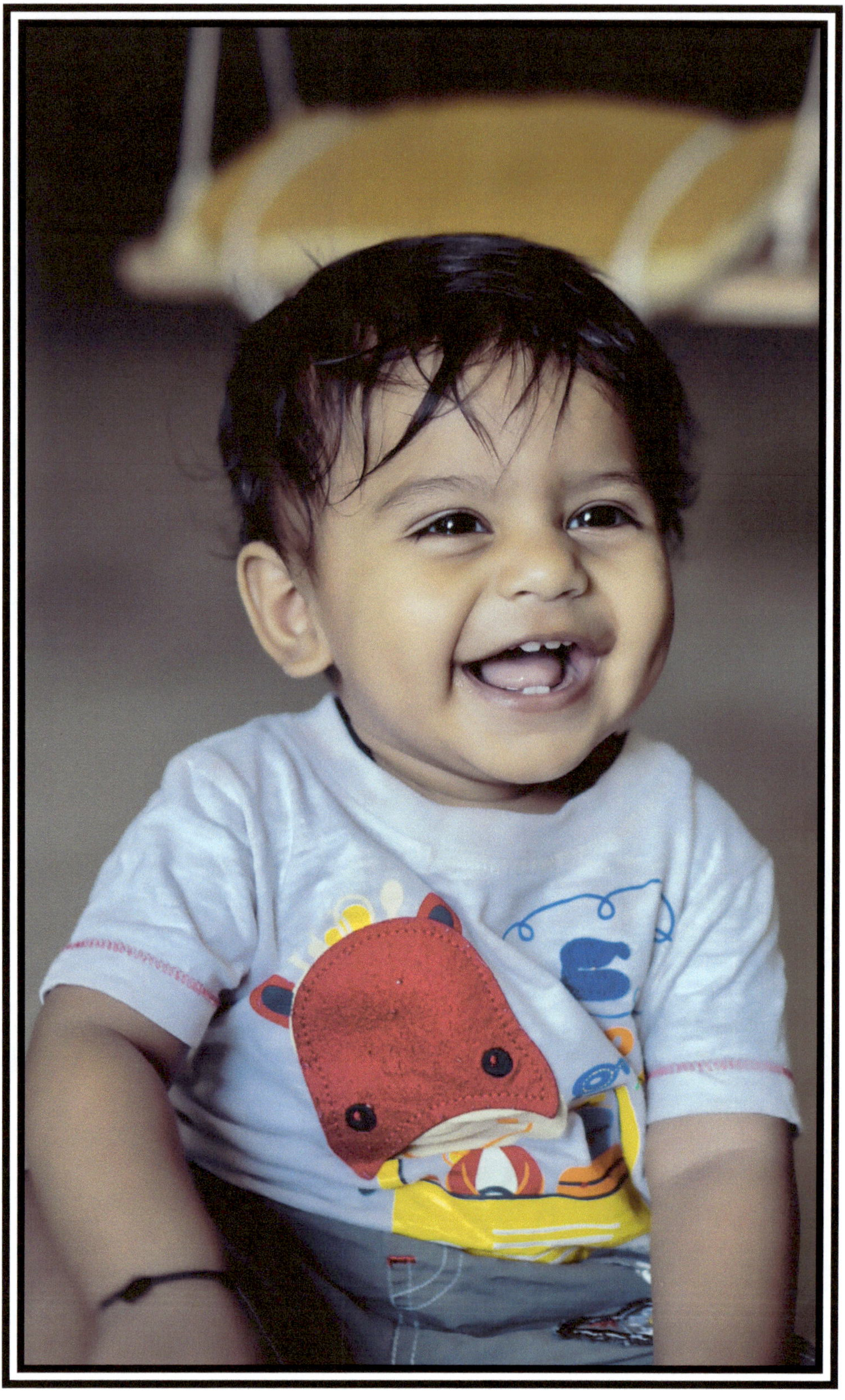

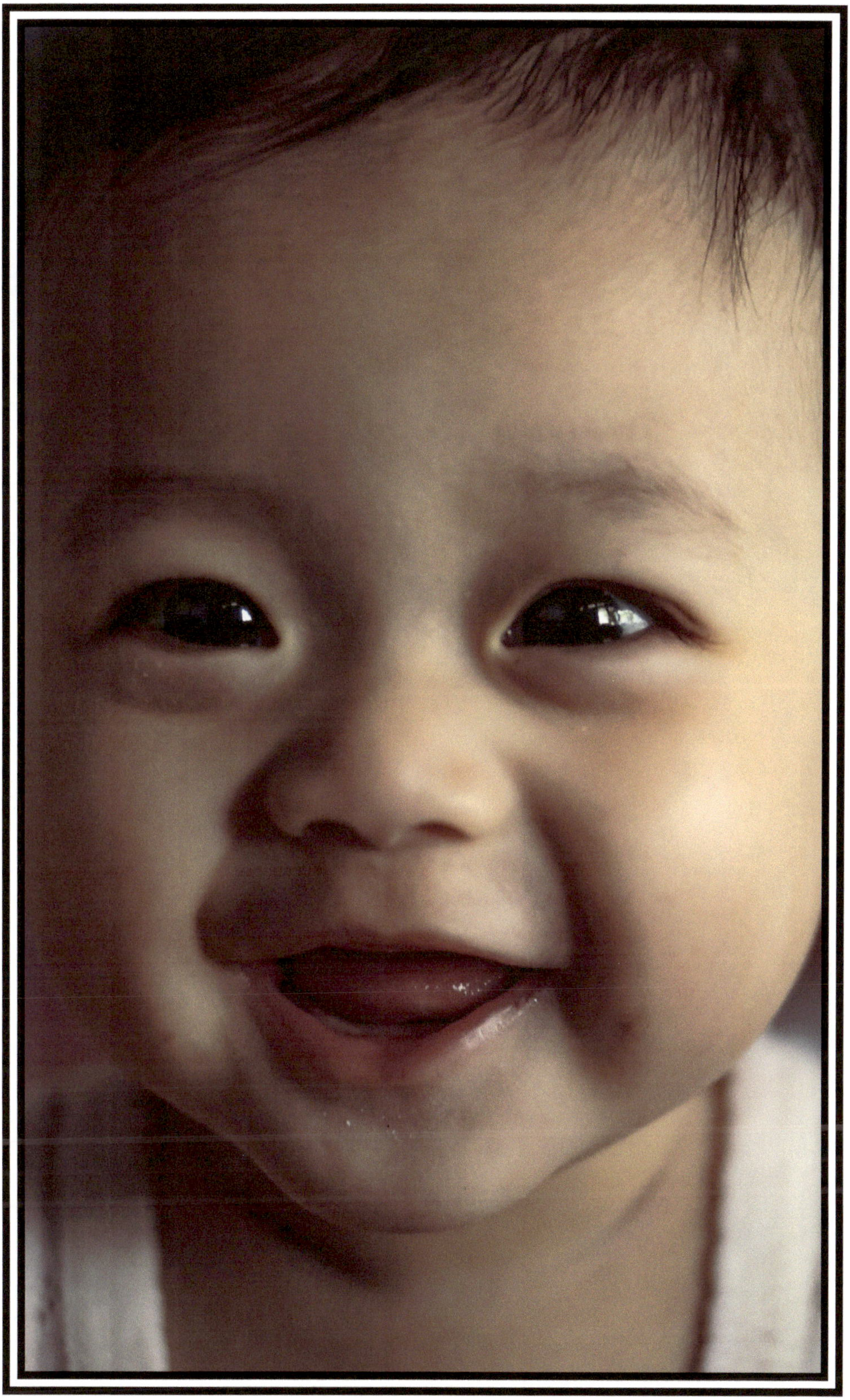

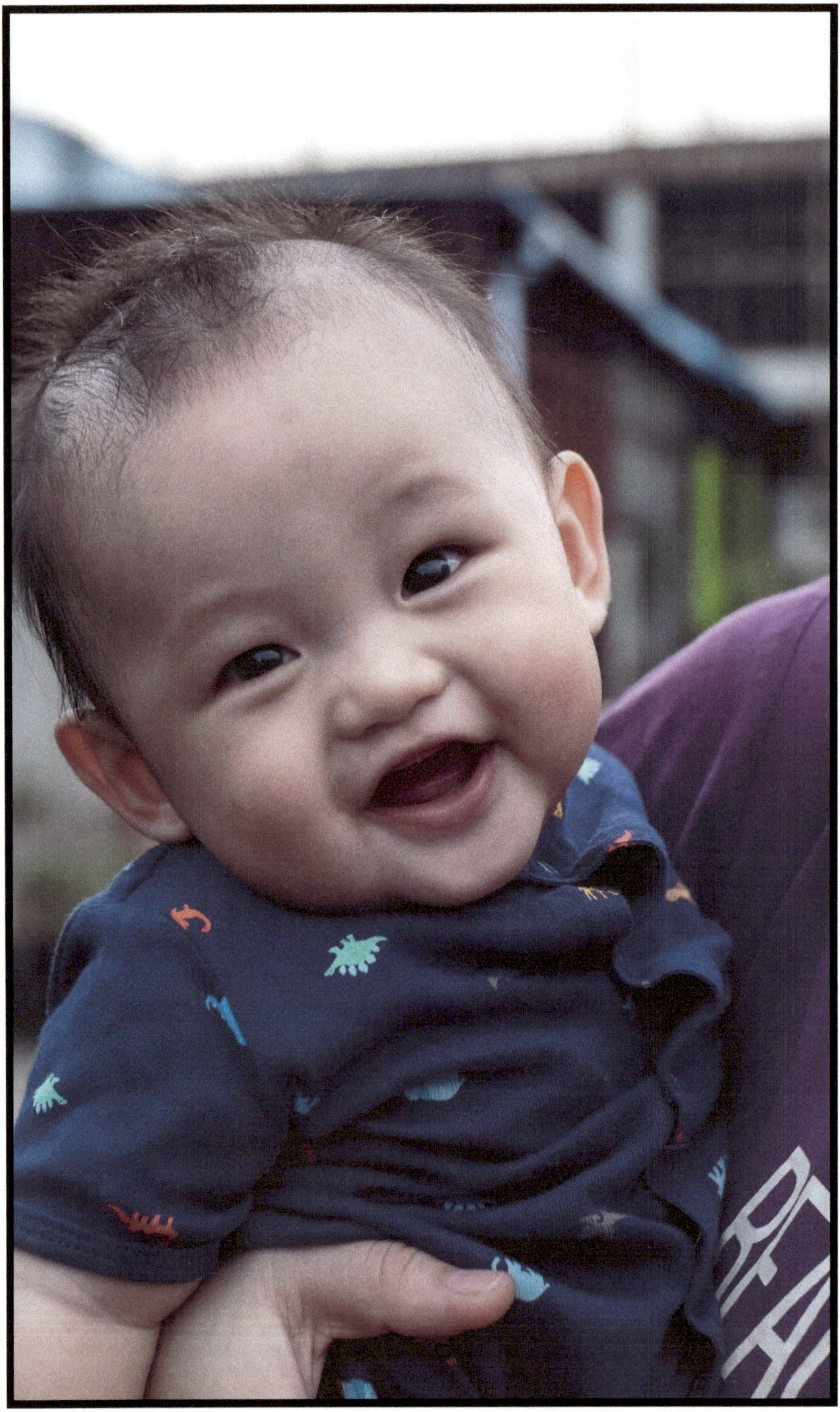

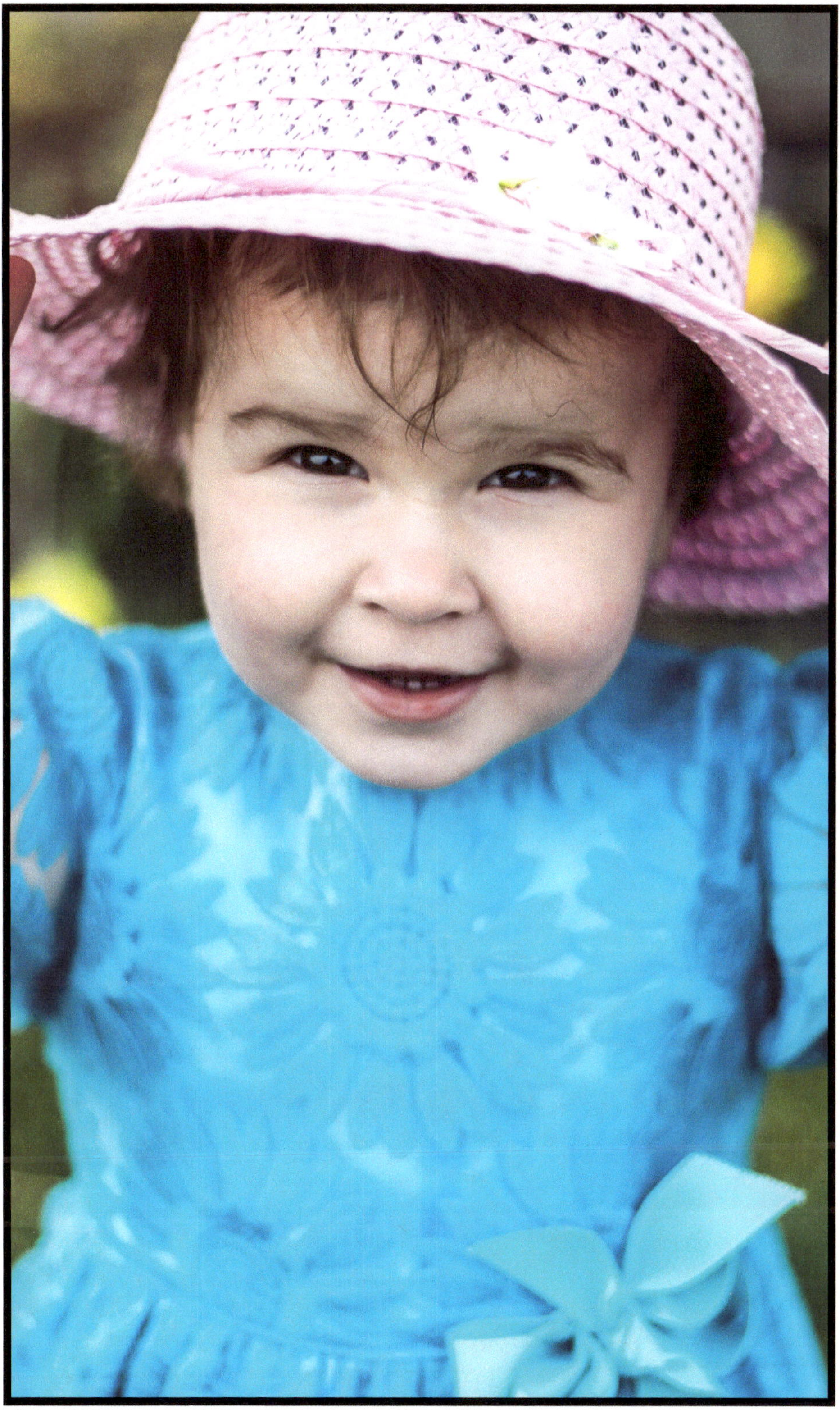

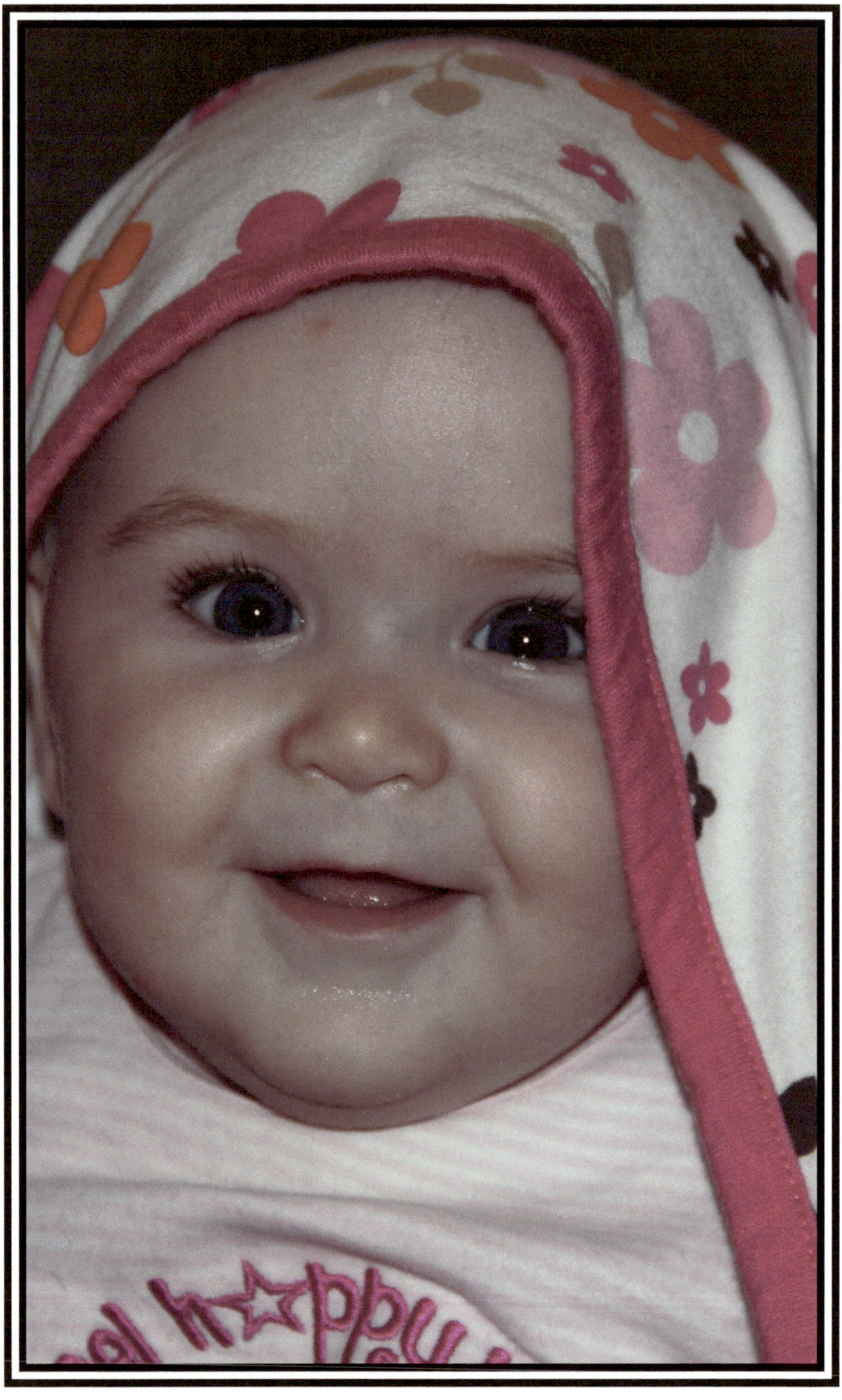

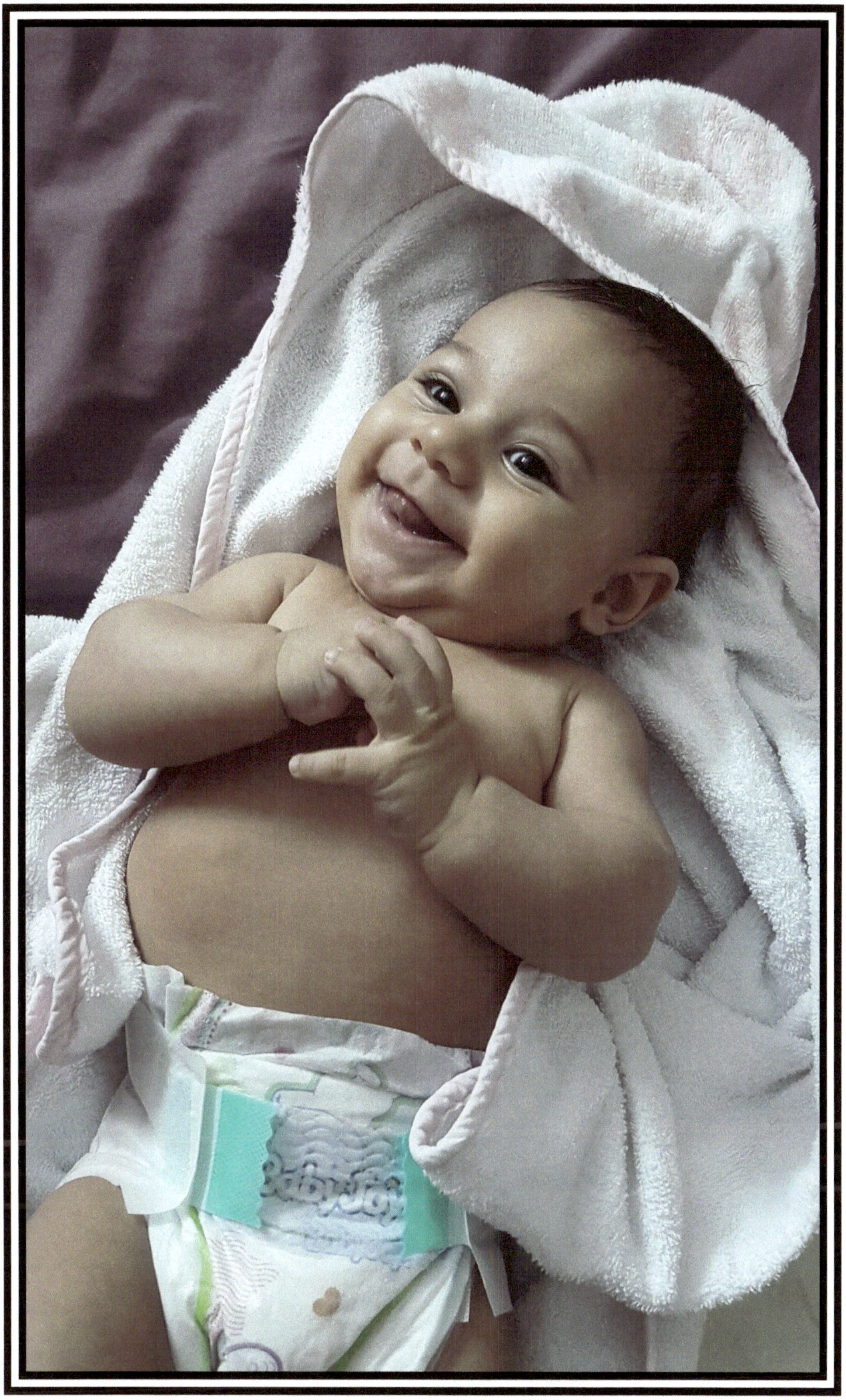

www.ingramcontent.com/pod-product-compliance
Lightning Source LLC
Chambersburg PA
CBHW040336220526
45473CB00009B/2707
* 9 7 9 8 5 7 7 9 7 3 4 0 7 *